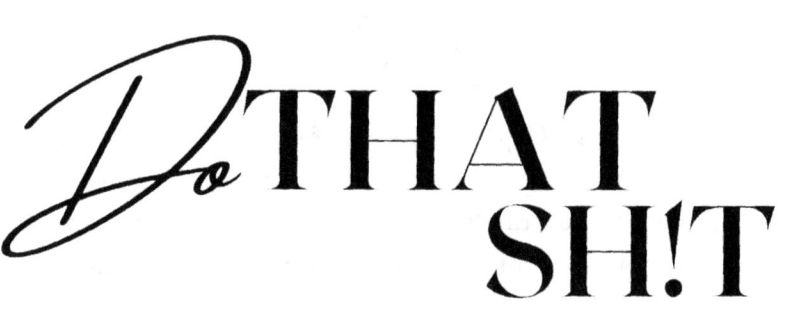

A Self-Rediscovery Journal

ASHLEY BRITTNEY SILVA

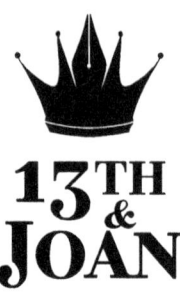

Do That Sh!t. Copyright 2022 by Ashley Brittney Silva. All rights reserved. No part of this publication may be reproduced, distributed, or transmitted in any form or by any means, including photocopying, recording, or other electronic or mechanical methods, without the prior written permission of the publisher, except in the case of brief quotations embodied in critical reviews and certain other noncommercial uses permitted by copyright law.

For permission requests, write to the publisher, addressed "Attention: Permissions Coordinator," 205 N. Michigan Avenue, Suite #810, Chicago, IL 60601. 13th & Joan books may be purchased for educational, business or sales promotional use. For information, please email the Sales Department at sales@13thandjoan.com.

Printed in the U. S. A.

First Printing, September 2022.

Library of Congress Cataloging-in-Publication Data has been applied for.

Paperback ISBN: 978-1-7326464-6-9
Hardcover ISBN: 978-1-953156-81-5

Dedication

THIS JOURNAL IS DEDICATED TO THE MOST BEAUTIFUL GIRL in the world, my daughter, Ashton. I am constantly inspired by the little lady you are at just 9 years old. Your compassion for others, your sass, your willingness to help others, your dedication to dance, the way that you support your friends (yasssss Queen), your random hugs, your encouragement, and the immeasurable confidence that you have in yourself pushes me to be a better person and woman.

I love you more than you love me, and that's on PERIOD. And ain't nothing after PERIOD.

(P.S. I'm sorry for all the bad words in this book.)

Dear Fear,

I've missed so much because of you. It won't happen again.

Acknowledgments

I WOULD LIKE TO THANK MY FAMILY! MY CHILDREN, ANTONIO and Ashton, I'm so blessed that God chose me for you. You are my purpose and my saving grace. Thank you to my husband, Quick, for being my biggest motivator and teacher. You've taught me that being a hustler is the only way to go and that I have everything in me that I need to succeed: hard work, dedication, and consistency! Mom, one of my biggest goals in life has always been to make you proud of me for simply being me. I hope that I've succeeded. To my sister, Tanesha (Pooh), thank you for being the best role model. WWPD? Thank you to my nieces, Diamond and Shaniya, for being the first loves of my life. To my godparents and my godsiblings, Sahara, Trenae, Tia, and Kevin, for being my very first audiences, whether it was my telling you about the latest celebrity news as a kid, making up song and dance routines, attending fashion shows, or us playing Apollo and Uno all summer break. Blood wouldn't make us any closer. Alicia, thank you for always being there, besides those two years that we didn't know each other. You are the definition of Ride or Die, a best friend, a sister. Katryce, thank you for your support and for coming into my life when I needed a friend like you the most. Cimon, your strength, support, and loyalty are unmatched. Ricky, my day one, my brother, thank you for always encouraging me. Angela, thank you for helping with everything from the kids to my website or just being a soundboard. Kendria, Dave, and Andrea thank you for always giving me an added boost of confidence when I needed it. To all my friends throughout my journey, for all the life lessons we've experienced, they all shaped me to be the person I am today. And a major thank you to everyone who has supported me in all of my many endeavors over the years. You all have shown me that I'm not someone who can be placed in a box..

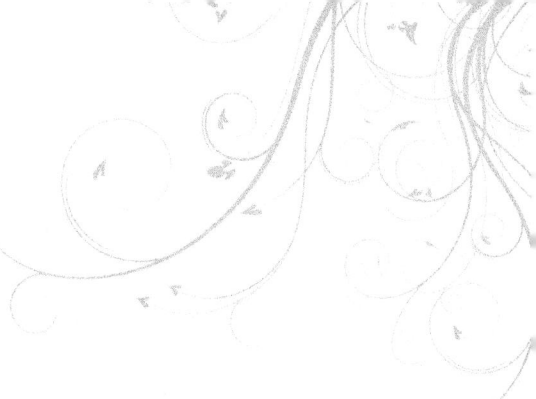

Disclaimer:
I CUSS A LITTLE BIT.

Y OU'VE BEEN WARNED. HEAL AT YOUR OWN RISK.
Before you begin, know that this book is the byproduct of unapologetic manifestation. For once in my life, I discovered the courage, freedom, and most importantly the peace to do something for myself, exactly the way that I wanted to do it.

While it is true that outward appearances suggest to many that I have been living my best life, nothing could be further from the truth. I, like many women, have spent years trapped. I was held hostage by who I thought I was supposed to be, who the world told me I should be, and the traumatized little girl I had suffocated for far too long. It was not until a few years ago that I decided to take my life and my future into my own hands, and along that journey, I discovered I was not alone.

Here's the hard truth that many are afraid to acknowledge: Women suffer in silence.

Through facing this reality, I learned that I had to put myself first. What does that mean? Putting yourself first means that you recognize you must fill your pitcher before pouring from it into others' cups. Let me also address the fact that putting yourself first does not mean to the detriment of others.

For much of my life, my pitcher remained empty until I realized that something needed to change. This is my journey in learning self-love, how to heal, and finally fulfill my dreams. Through this story, I wish to give you the means to do the same. Read the journal prompts and affirmations provided, and take the time to reflect on your journey.

Let us start to fill your cup. Self-love and getting what you want out of life comes solely from you, not others.

This book is for everyone and anyone. But as a woman, a Black woman, I want to affirm this message: Too often women are told to be confident, but not too confident. Told to use their voice, but don't be too loud. Told to be what and who they want as long as it fits into what society deems acceptable. FUCK THAT! DO WHAT YOU WANT. DO THAT SHIT!

Contents

Dedication vii

Acknowledgments ix

It Takes A Village 3

How I Got Here 21

Dear Village 35

Who the Fuck are You? 41

Revelation 53

Reflection 61

The First Step to Change is to Become Aware of Your Own Bullshit! 73

Be Proud of Who You Are Instead of Ashamed of Who You Aren't. 81

Heal That Shit 103

Realization 133

The Work 149

Set Limits in Your Life 167

A Hobby and Self-care	173
Fuck That Shit	177
Taking Time Off For Me	183
Do the Fucking Work	189
You Deserve That Shit	195
Epilogue	201

ASHLEY BRITTNEY SILVA

Journal Prompt #1: On a day when you are feeling on top of the world, like the baddest bitch that ever walked this earth, looking good and feeling better, make a list of 20 things (or more because you're a baddie) that you love about yourself and your life. And on the days you are feeling shitty or less than a baddie, pull that list out, look in the mirror, and read that list out loud.

1. _____

2. _____

3. _____

4. _____

5. _____

6. _____

7. _____

8. _____

9. _____

DO THAT SH!T

10. _____

11. _____

12. _____

13. _____

14. _____

15. _____

16. _____

17. _____

18. _____

19. _____

20. _____

It Takes A Village

How many times have you thought to yourself, "I wish that time would slow down. That everything could just stop. Stop, so that I could figure out my life, my next steps, or what my purpose is?"

For me, that wish was granted in March 2020. The world stopped (Beyoncé voice)! COVID-19 swept the globe and forced most of us to take a seat from the hustle and bustle of our everyday lives. This gave us the wildly requested present of time. It may not have come packaged as nice and neatly as we had hoped for but, like Aladdin and the Genie, wish granted. We were stripped to the bare necessities and left with only time to prepare for our new norm, which hopefully included getting things previously put on the back burner done.

Journal Prompt #2: What did you do with the time given to you during COVID-19?

ASHLEY BRITTNEY SILVA

Outside of the selfless essential workers, many of us spent our quarantine binge-watching TV, getting in some much-needed cleaning, napping, partying to DJs on Instagram Live, spending countless hours on TikTok, attending Zoom meetings, meditating, praying, and doing at-home workouts. Then throw in the scarcity of toilet paper, cleaning products, hand sanitizer, face masks, gloves, the anxiety of grocery shopping, and homeschooling our kids with a glass or five of wine. Many of these things were a much-needed wake-up call to what had become our daily need to be busy. As if busy, successful, and productive are synonyms of one another. They are not.

Journal Prompt #3: How many of you took advantage of your much requested, "I need more time to get to all of the things I have been wanting to do for years, but just can not find the time to do it" done? Did you maximize the time? What do you wish you had done differently?

_____

_____

_____

_____

_____

_____

_____

_____

_____

_____

_____

_____

_____

Before we go any further let me tell you all a little about myself and why I decided to write this journal. I am Ashley Silva, born and raised on the west side of Baltimore, Maryland. I grew up being book smart, and because of the neighborhood that I was raised in and many of the life situations I faced, street smart too. I am a mom, wife, daughter, sister, aunt, friend, and so much more. I have read dozens of self-help books–some useful, some redundant, many boring, but not too many that truly elicit raw emotional reactions. No book told me exactly what was wrong and how to fix it, and especially there was no book that unlocked my deeply buried trauma and emotions. So, after a five-year journey to rediscover myself and finally feel hopeful, and dare I say happy, I decided that I needed to write my own "mind-opening" and "spiritual awakening" story that allows people like me to finally pick up a book that could truly change their lives.

Journal Prompt #4: The late, great Maya Angelou once said, "People do not grow up…they get older." Let that quote sit with you. What does it mean to you?

_____
_____
_____
_____
_____
_____
_____
_____
_____
_____
_____
_____
_____
_____
_____

Age and maturity are not the same. We can live to be 100 years old, with all the wrinkles to match, yet we can mentally remain stagnant. Without mentally maturing we are simply vessels of old age. When I reflected on my life, I realized that I was merely growing older. The years went by, and the birthdays came and went, but my soul was only growing weary and tired.

I have been exactly where you are. I was completely lost with what my purpose in life was. I mean, I thought I knew what my purpose was, but as the candles filled the birthday cakes, I lost faith in myself, my hopes, and my dreams. For so long, too long, I was unhappy and struggling with so much of my own shit that I felt like I was drowning in it.

I thought by this age I would have reached my lifelong dreams of starring in a handful of movies and TV shows, and that I would now be the host of my own daytime talk show. But that wasn't the case. I barely graduated high school after missing one too many days. Truthfully, a lot of days. I did not go directly to a traditional college like most of my friends. At 18 I was working full time, had bought my first car, and was helping with household bills. By 23 I was a wife, mom, and homeowner. I dabbled in and out of colleges with a list of completed psychology and fashion courses as well as certifications earned in broadcasting and makeup artistry, but I was floating through life with no true direction. Since 2010, I have had two blogs and an online radio show. I currently have a podcast and lifestyle brand called *Fun Time Moms*, a community for today's mothers navigating through parenthood. Over the years, I have helped many of my listeners and social media followers traverse their lives with my transparency and advice.

I live in a nice house and drive a nice car. My Instagram page consists of a decent following, with pictures of my smiling face, some cute outfits, my family, friends, and a few celebrities here and there. On the outside looking in I was living the new American dream. But on the inside, I was empty as hell. I felt every "un" possible there is. Unfulfilled, unaccomplished, unmotivated, unloved.

    I never felt like I was living the life I saw for myself when I was a young girl. I was *just* a wife and a mom with a pretty mundane routine. I would wake up, get the kids ready for school, go home, clean up, wash clothes, pick up the kids after school, do basketball and dance drop-offs, cook dinner, sleep, and repeat.

    All of my aspirations were seemingly slipping away.

Journal Prompt #5: Be honest with your current self. Are you truly where you've always wanted to be? Do you feel any "uns" like I had? List them out.

When my now-husband and I seriously started dating, I was 20 years old with a full-time job, working in an office at a furniture store. I had just bought a Lexus flat out with cash. Sooner than later it died on me, and I then got a Hyundai that I affectionately named Sky. Still, the best car I have ever had. I was fresh out of broadcasting school and pursuing a career in broadcast entertainment. My now-husband was a well-known local DJ and radio personality with a career that was skyrocketing. As soon as I turned 21, I landed a job in promotions with a talk/sports radio station. Not the type of station I saw myself at, but it was a foot in the door, and I was excited. My duties were to set up at local bars and any other of the station's events. Only two months in I found out that I was pregnant. I was newly 21, pregnant, and early in my first serious relationship as an adult. I honestly didn't know what I wanted to do. I never saw myself as a young mother, and I felt my dreams of stardom would be over once I became one.

Since my now-husband was also pushing toward his career, I thought he'd feel the same—that a baby would derail his career, but he was so excited to start a family. I was afraid and young, but we moved along and prepared to have a child.

I tried to keep working, but the job required a lot from me. Lifting was heavy, and I was
always exhausted. I would be in the club until 2 a.m. with drunk sports fans, and that was not
really the place for a pregnant woman, so I quit.

I was 21, watching my friends be young, free 21-year-old's living their lives, going out, partying, and getting their degrees. I was home alone and expecting a baby. My husband was working 10 to 15-hour days. I was constantly lonely, yearning for a life I watched others around me so freely live. There were days that I felt like a bug caught in a web of circumstances that I feared would force me to lose my life. Shortly after my son's birth, we moved a little over an hour away from my family and friends. Isolation became my new normal.

Journal Prompt #6: Are there circumstances you are currently facing that are affecting your daily life? Your goals? How do they make you feel?

_____

_____

_____

_____

_____

_____

_____

_____

_____

_____

_____

_____

_____

_____

Once my son was a year old, I enrolled him in a childcare center and went back to school. I convinced myself that I needed to put my dreams of having a career in broadcasting behind me. It was a demanding career that wasn't going to wait around for me or anyone else to get a babysitter. I decided to pursue something else that I found enjoyable–fashion. I felt this was a career I could do while being a mom that would not require too much time away from my son. For a while, things were going well. I enrolled in school majoring in fashion merchandising with a 4.0 GPA, but I was soon hit with another blow. I had to take a required class that overlapped with my son's pick-up time from daycare. The roadblock I faced was a mountain I could not climb. My husband was always working, and I didn't have anyone close by who could get my son and watch him for a few hours. We had just bought our first single-family home, so money was tight, and a nanny was out of the question. I had to drop out of school. There was no conversation about it or plan of action to find me help. It was over.

I was then 23. No degree. No job. Sad as hell. Just a mom. Just a wife.

I felt like a failure. This was not the life that I planned for myself. To not have my career. To not achieve my own goals. To be a kept woman. To have to depend on my husband 100 percent financially. I had to ask my husband for money whenever I needed anything and everything. I started to resent him. Nothing had changed in his life since we had become parents. His career was flourishing. He was in high demand, and it seemed like every week he was presented with a great new opportunity. I was jealous. I resented him. I hated myself. I hated my life.

For years I lived this way. When I say years, I mean over a decade. I sat every day with the feeling of anger toward my situation. I was never given a choice. Never consulted or considered. I was a mom, and that was all people expected me to be. So many women are expected to lose themselves within their status as a mother. Taking care of your child should be your only job, and if it is not, then you have to try extra hard to show that you can still be a good mother while working. The woman behind the mother disappears within herself. My husband worked extremely hard to provide a good life for our family, and I didn't complain for fear of seeming ungrateful, but my needs ceased to be met outside of material things.

    Over that decade of feeling lost and alone, I had another baby. A few years after the birth of my daughter I over-exhausted myself with my first blog, I Am SuperGorge, and had a mental breakdown. I knew that I had to make a change in my life, seek help, and move in a different direction to save myself.

Journal Prompt #7: If you are a mother, have you ever been able to relate to my experiences of feeling lonely and placed on the back burner? If you are not in the role of mother, what circumstances or situations create these feelings in you?

_____

_____

_____

_____

_____

_____

_____

_____

_____

_____

_____

_____

_____

_____

Journal Prompt #8: Have others neglected your personal needs, goals, and desires? Have you neglected yourself?

_____

_____

_____

_____

_____

_____

_____

_____

_____

_____

_____

_____

_____

_____

_____

AFFIRMATIONS:

- [ ] I am important.
- [ ] I am valuable.
- [ ] My goals and dreams are worthy of being attained.
- [ ] My needs deserve to be met.

How I Got Here

I HAVE GONE THROUGH THE MAJORITY OF MY LIFE NOT feeling good enough. Not good enough for my parents, my husband, my family, and my friends. I felt like everyone hated me and simply tolerated me. My parents were divorced when I was 3. I have no memory of ever being in a two-parent household or seeing a loving, happy marriage. Growing up, I would see my dad on some weekends. Those, however, were few and far between. He remarried and moved to another state when I was about 7 or 8. I had gone to visit for about two weeks in the summer, but it was clear his wife and new family were his priority, not me.

One summer while visiting–I call it the "Cinderella Summer"– my two stepsisters had me get on a bike with no brakes, unbeknownst to me, and go down a long steep country road. That bike ride ended with two permanent scars, both of which I still have, five stitches on my chin, and a vow that I would never go back there another summer. I kept my promise and never did. That was pretty much the end of our already fragile father-daughter relationship.

Journal Prompt #9: What was your relationship like with your parents as a child? Has that relationship changed as you've grown older?

My mom always told me that as a young child I was attached to her hip, a memory I do not remember. I do not recall being mommy's mini-me or little princess. Once I was a teenager, I felt like my mother resented me for my dad not being there. Resented me for being so outspoken and opinionated. She resented having to raise me alone, unlike she had to do with my older sister, who my grandmother raised. That sense of resentment for me was rooted deep within our relationship. I've always known that my mother loves me, but that love too often felt like it was hampered by disappointments and came with conditions that were utterly beyond my control.

Journal Prompt #10: Have you ever felt like your parents' love had conditions? Does that kind of love impact you to this day?

During my childhood, I was at my grandmother's house a lot. My school and my friends were there. I was there. By the time I was in the 7th grade, my grandmother passed away from cancer. I watched as my grandmother took her final breath in her hospital bed, an image forever embedded in my mind. My mom was left with an outspoken, bullheaded, 13-year-old to raise completely by herself, something she never had to do before. From there, our relationship went downhill.

There were never any shopping dates, no mommy and me mani-pedis. There were always disagreements and arguments. At 16, right after getting my driver's license at the end of my junior year of high school, my mom met a man and moved out. I remember her packing her overnight bag and stuffing it with her belongings like she was running away. I watched her back as she walked out the door, bag in hand, and never came back. I was 16 and alone.

I let all my responsibility fall by the wayside. There was no adult to keep me in check, so I started partying and hanging out all hours of the night. It was summer, and I was having a ball. There wasn't much harm done until fall when I started my senior year of high school. For a few months, I would get up and drive myself to school every day. Then after a while, I skipped a day or two here and there and then a week, two weeks…a month. I simply stopped going to school.

During that time I also had a huge blow-up with a close friend over a simple misunderstanding. She believed that I had abandoned her when she'd gotten a flat tire. The blow-up resulted in her hitting me and, of course, our friendship ended. The harsh break-up and my mother not being home with me caused me to feel so alone. I already had more than enough credits to graduate from high school, so I wanted to move on. I was over all of it.

Over high school, over my high school friends, and over being a kid. I retaliated out of anger and pain and from there I went into full party mode.

My mom will tell you that I was mature for my age and that my older sister was living with me at the time. In reality, I was a little girl who looked kind of like a grown woman on the outside, but on the inside, I was hurting and feeling abandoned. My sister was barely 24 and had two small children of her own when she moved back in eight months after my mom moved out. She was in no way capable of raising a 16-year-old. For over a decade I was so angry with my mother. Angry at her for choosing a man over me. Angry for her not being there in the mornings to make sure I was off to high school. Pissed at her that I didn't go straight to college.

Looking back, I see how my relationship with my mother and my friend molded me moving forward. I over-compensated and over-worried. I never wanted anyone else I cared for to think I had left them stranded, in need, or wouldn't be there for them, so I began to overextend myself. I made sure that I was always there anytime I was needed. Even within my marriage, I pursued my husband first. He didn't have to chase or win me over. I have loved him since I met him. You know the saying, "Marry someone who loves you more than you love them?" Well, I felt my husband did that. Ouch, that one stings. But it is my truth and as I have said we are here for honesty, transparency, and uncovering those harsh realities.

Journal Prompt #11: How have your past relationships impacted the way you seek and give love to your current ones?

Living the way that I had left me feeling depleted. I never felt back all the love I was so freely giving, and desperately wanted in return. I rarely even felt liked. I felt replaceable and that I was simply existing and being tolerated by everyone in my life. What I now realize is that all of that love that I was so freely giving away was me seeking someone or something that would return it the same way. I was desperately hoping someone would see my value and pour it into me.

The truth is, I didn't love myself. My pitcher was empty. I gave nothing to myself because I did not believe that I deserved it. I was putting huge expectations on people hoping they would see me, love me, and not simply take from me. I thought I needed their validation, but I didn't. I still do not. Others are not qualified to validate me. In reality, what I gave away to others should have been saved for myself. I deserved to value myself as much as I valued those around me.

Now in my 30s, I see that the expectations I placed on others were impossible for them to meet as well. I have realized that it must have been extremely hard for my mother to go from having full-time help and support from my grandmother to having to raise a teenager on her own for the first time, all while grieving the loss of her mother. Now that I have my children I realize that as a mom sometimes it feels like it is all too much to handle. My mother saw a way out and took it. As a teenager, I should have gotten myself up to go to high school. I knew better. I will not make excuses for my mother, but I do understand her actions better now. Sometimes by walking in someone else's shoes, you can help explain their actions, even understand them, without having to excuse them. Empathy and forgiveness are vital in learning to heal your trauma and continue your journey.

I was upset with my mother for not loving me right, upset with my father for not being there for me, and upset with my friends for discrediting me. I was angry because it felt like everyone had abandoned me, but I knew that I had to learn to heal from that pain as well. The first step was to recognize that I allowed that trauma and those people to change me and my goals. I had to take accountability for my actions and forgive everyone else who I had been blaming for years. Some fucked-up things had happened to me, but I put my entire self-worth in the hands of others. They did not have to love me the way I wanted them to. It was not their responsibility.

Now do not get me wrong. I wholeheartedly believe in reciprocal relationships of all kinds. But we cannot put these huge demands and expectations on others, letting what they do or do not do define us. Ultimately, we need to do what we need to do to take control of our own lives and accept people for who they are, flaws and all–the same way that I want to be accepted as flawed as I am.

Journal Prompt #12: Who in your life can you practice empathy with that you have not been able to before? Can you recognize their wrongdoings while also recognizing their humanity?

Journal Prompt #13: Have there been times when you have allowed others to take control of your fate? What part of those moments or paths can you take ownership for?

I have also learned that while I was forgiving others, I had to do the same for myself. Over time, I learned to forgive myself for not knowing better and for not doing better. This took not only time but maturity.

Aaliyah said it best, *"Age Ain't Nothing But A Number."*

Our age does not make us mature or healthy mentally. What makes us mature is being able to have real and raw conversations with ourselves about ourselves. I had to learn to peel back the layers and face my own shit. It was not an overnight process, and even now I have realized that the process of healing is an ongoing one. I still have bad days. Healing is a choice I make daily. I have gone from hating the soul of the person I saw in the mirror to learning to accept the person I am. Dare I say, I may be falling deeply in love with her ass. This has been learned through years of heartbreak, forgiveness, failing, being overlooked, being misunderstood, understanding others, therapy, forming safe circles, medication, meditation, and my self-determination to do that shit. I want to achieve and live my life on my terms, no matter what it looks like to anyone else. I decided to let go of all the BS excuses I had used in the past that held me back.

There was a time not too long ago that I never thought I would get here, but here I am, and if I can do it, so can you. There is nothing that I am asking of you that I have not or do not require of myself. I may not be everything I want to be, but every day I am more than I was yesterday. That is progress. We control the trajectory of our lives. Hop off of the hamster wheel. You are capable and more than enough. The life you desire and deserve is waiting for you. It is time for you to do that shit.

Journal Prompt #14: What steps can you take to begin your journey to a better you? Think therapy, personal health, relationship work, career change, and/or so much more.

AFFIRMATIONS:

- [ ] I am human, and I make mistakes.
- [ ] My mistakes do not define me.
- [ ] I am in control of my life.
- [ ] I will no longer make excuses.
- [ ] I will learn to forgive those around me.
- [ ] I will learn to forgive myself.

Dear Village

Throughout this self-rediscovery journal, I will share a lot about my life with you. If any of what I share feels familiar to you, then you picked up the right journal. Maybe your life is not exactly where mine was, but you know you want, need, and deserve more. Right now, you may feel as though you are constantly trying but steadily hitting roadblocks. You may feel that no matter how hard you work, it goes unnoticed. You may be unhappy in your current situation, whether it is your job, your health, your weight, your relationship, living arrangements, or your financial situation. What you want feels so unattainable. I am here to tell you it is not. You can have the life you want.

By the end of this journal, you will be able to understand your struggles and push through them, not just get around them or over them. You will believe that you are worthy of what you've been asking for. You are going to look back on the person you used to be. You will forgive yourself for not knowing better. You will hug yourself and know that everything will be ok because you have decided to push past the shit that has kept you stuck and go after what you want for yourself and your life. You will dream bigger and achieve more than you ever believed was possible. You will have awakened the tools that are already buried inside you to take your life to the next level.

The process is necessary, but it is not pretty.

You see, this is not for the person who is looking to be perfect and have every box on the list checked. Perfection does not exist. It is bullshit. This is for the person who does not have all their shit together, coming from a woman who does not have all her shit together and is perfectly OK with that. In life, we all have challenges. What we must learn is not how to avoid challenges but how to successfully navigate through them and take the lessons that come with them. In the instances where you cannot change your circumstances, you must learn to make them work for you.

I am not going to coddle you on this journey to self-rediscovery. I will not hold your hand through this process, but I will hold you accountable and have your back. What we are about to get into is real work. *Hard work.*

This is not just a journal on how to manifest and positively think yourself into your dream life. Those things are important, and we will do them, but there is so much more to getting what you want out of life. You have to do the fucking work. Every single day. Not just when you feel like it.

You will want to cry. You will want to hide from this journal and yourself. You will want to say, "Who TF does she think she is telling me what to do?" You'll want to quit—again. But you've done all of those things before and where has it gotten you?

This time around, I want you to stick it out and take a chance on yourself. No more hiding and denying yourself real happiness. What's the worst thing that could happen? You achieve your dreams?

Maybe you will land your dream job. Maybe you will finally start your business. Maybe you will buy that house. Maybe you will lose those 10 pounds. Maybe you will finish your degree or get your master's. Maybe you will adopt that child or get married. Or just maybe, you will fall in love with your life.

It is time to rediscover who you really are and DO THAT SHIT!

Journal Prompt #15: Make a list of all of your current goals. Write beside them how you plan to achieve them. Number your goals by how important they are to you. Do your actions to achieve your goals align with their importance to you?

AFFIRMATIONS:

- [ ] I am resilient.
- [ ] I make no excuses.
- [ ] I am good enough.

Who the Fuck are You?

LIKE MOST OF YOU, IF SOMEONE ASKED ME "WHO ARE YOU?" I would tell them my name, followed by family and job titles. But that is not WHO I am. That is WHAT I do. Very often I meet people and they say, "Oh you are QuickSilva's wife." Yes, I am, but have they forgotten that I am also a person outside of that? Whenever I show up to school or extra-curricular activities, I am simply "Antonio's mom" or "Ashton's mom."

Honestly, after about a decade of being a mom and wife, I did not know who the fuck I was anymore. I knew who I was pretending to be, who I had convinced myself I should be, who others expected me to be, but I had lost myself. It seemed like every day a piece of me chipped away. I appeared confident to others, but I hated everything about myself. I hated my appearance, big nose, dark circles, my height, my weight, my big feet, and so much more.

I hated that I was always sad and angry. Why couldn't I just be happy? I thought of myself as a good mom, wife, and friend, but that didn't make me feel accomplished. I craved more out of my life. I hated that I had not achieved anything in my adulthood that

I was proud of. These feelings persisted despite my mother often telling me that she is proud of me. Since I have had deep-rooted insecurities for decades, all positive feelings toward myself have been hindered by self-doubt. What was she so proud of?

    Growing up, I had super high expectations placed on me. I was super confident. The smart, talkative, outgoing, most likely-to-succeed type of child. My mom always tells a story of how I started talking the day I came home from the hospital. Due to my know-it-all attitude and never backing down from an argument my mother thought I was going to be a lawyer, and no little girl wants to disappoint their mommy. So for years, whenever the question was asked, that is what I said I wanted to be when I grew up. From that moment on my mom was convinced that was what I was going to do with my life. Being an attorney is an amazing career choice, and I do think that I would have been good at it, but even at 5 years old I knew that was not what I wanted to do with my life.

Journal Prompt #16: Have you ever had any big expectations placed on you as a child? How did that impact the way you saw your failures or life goal changes?

My dreams were of stardom! Being a girl from west Baltimore, wanting a life of stardom might have seemed far-fetched, but it wasn't for me. It was my destiny. There was a time when I finally saw that destiny become reality for someone else and it suddenly didn't seem so far away. I was sitting home watching *A Different World* when a new character was introduced to the show. Her name was Lena James, a girl from Baltimore. In real life that cute, petite girl dressed in hip-hop clothes was Jada Pinkett, a girl from Baltimore, just like me. She was not the cookie-cutter image that had been painted by Hollywood. She reminded me of so many girls I had seen in my day-to-day life, and she was the motivation that I needed. If she could do it, so could I.

Journal Prompt #17: Who or what in your life has been your greatest inspiration and motivation? Have you had any celebrities or people in your life that you have looked up to?

As a child, I knew that one purpose in my life was to work in entertainment. Way before blogs and social media, I could give you a rundown of celebrities' lives. I knew all the pop culture drama and news. I was into all the latest movies, music, TV shows, and magazines. Not only did I dream big, I knew exactly what I wanted to do with my life by the time I was 10. Being a lawyer was my mom's dream for me, not my own. Without a doubt, I had a dream career that mirrored Oprah Winfrey's. I wanted to be a talk show host, actress, and magazine owner. I would live out my dreams in real life as a young girl. If there was a school play, I was in it. I made up songs and dance routines with my godsisters and friends during all of our sleepovers. When my mom wasn't home, I would go into her closet and put on her fancy clothes, do my makeup, and practice in the mirror for hours doing interviews with myself. Aside from plays in elementary school, in middle school I was in the drama club, and in high school I earned my International Baccalaureate Certification in Theater. There was not a doubt in my mind that I would follow in the footsteps of my hometown hero. I had found my passion in entertainment.

But as time went on, my support system seemed to be a party of one, and I lost that strong belief in myself. I did not go straight to college but still wanted to pursue my dreams of acting and broadcasting. My mom's high hopes for Ashley, Esq., were gone. Whenever I talked about my road to stardom, she would tell me to "stop living in a fantasy world," a statement that has echoed in my head every time I thought about taking a leap of faith. So instead of jetting off to Hollywood, I started working full time at 18. I figured I had to save up some money and then pursue my dreams. Over time I began doubting myself and my talent more and more.

With every bump that I hit in the road, I'd hear my mother's words echoing in my head, "You are living in a fantasy world."

Maybe she was right. Maybe I should have become a lawyer. At least if I was going to be unhappy in my career, I would have had a steady paycheck and a title that was deemed adequate by others.

Journal Prompt #18: Has anyone ever told you that your dreams or goals are unrealistic? Did that stop or discourage you from pursuing them?

Soon after I became a mom and wife, I decided to put fairy tales behind me. Although I still knew deep inside of myself that entertainment was my God-given talent, I tried to suppress my dreams.

In her book *Untamed*, Gwendolyn Doyls talks of people calling women "selfless" for continuously putting others first. "The epitome of womanhood is to lose oneself completely," she wrote. This quote hit me like a round of bullets.

I had lost myself completely trying to be the perfect mom and wife, trying to be the always-dependable friend so that I wasn't a good Ashley. I didn't even know who Ashley was anymore or what she wanted.

Now in my 30s, once I decided that I had to do what I needed to do for myself, my life changed. My zest for life has come back. I feel the most creative I have ever felt, and my passions burst through me. There are so many business ideas that I have, and I am finally finding reassurance in myself and my talents. Life has never felt so vivid. Though there are still days when I am filled with self-doubt, I work to center myself and trust in my plan.

Journal Prompt #19: How has what others expect from you impacted your dreams?

AFFIRMATIONS:

☐ What others think of me does not hold me back.
☐ My happiness is not flexible.

Revelation

Back in 2010, I decided to start putting myself out there as a blogger and interviewer with my first blog IAMSUPERGORGE.COM, an entertainment-based website with an emphasis on the everyday woman's life. I covered everything I loved from entertainment, beauty, and fashion to the modern-day millennial-raised family.

I contacted local party promoters to see if they had celebrities hosting their events and offered to promote their event in exchange for an interview. If I saw that a celebrity was going to be in my city, I would go on Twitter and Instagram to DM publicists, managers, and the talent themselves to request interviews. A lot of those emails and DMs went unanswered, but every once in a while I got a response. Many times I heard "no," but there were also opportunities that came with a "yes." I was able to interview stars like Kelly Rowland, Megan Good, Michael Ealy, and legends Chaka Khan and Dionne Warwick. I started to be invited as press to cover red-carpet events where prestigious media like *Essence* magazine were also attending as interviewers. I also had the opportunity to host true-crime TV shows. Looking from the outside in, others would think I am lucky and successful. That was only in their eyes. I often, even to this day, have an overwhelming sense of not being good enough for the place I am in. I was suffering from "imposter syndrome," which is defined as "not trusting in your abilities" or "feeling like a fraud." Yes, I went to broadcasting school, but I did not have a degree in journalism. Yes, I lived and breathed entertainment news, but I did not work for a well-known publication. So why was I here? Did I belong!?

Journal Prompt #20: Have you ever felt like an imposter? Write about it and how it made you feel.

The answer was "Hell yes!" I belonged right on those red carpets next to those big-name publications because that was and still is my calling! The same way that your grandmother who has never been to culinary school can put that restaurant down the street to shame is the same way I know entertainment. I had to let go of the imposter syndrome. I was not an imposter! I was exactly where I was supposed to be. Though I still struggle with it, now I can recognize that what I am feeling is not the truth. The truth is that you are good enough to be in that space just like I am. If you are there, then you are meant to be there.

I also learned to stop looking at myself as *just* a mom and wife. Being a mom and a wife, a good one–fuck that, a great one–is no easy task. If there is nothing else that I accomplished in my lifetime, the family that I have created is award-winning in my book. My children are amazing. They are healthy and extremely intelligent. They are pursuing things that they enjoy, but most importantly, my children know that they are deeply loved by me. When they are excited about something, I am the first person they want to tell. When they are hurt, sick, or sad, they curl up in my bed and lay on me just like they did as babies. Even my almost 15-year-old son who is now towering over me. I am their safe place. I am their home, and that is a huge accomplishment. For years I took this for granted because I felt like it was just what I was supposed to do. There was no thought put into it. But being a great mom is a game-changer. Just look at those who do not have those relationships with their parents. I am molding children who will eventually be extraordinary young adults, who will lead their lives with compassion for others, and who will be self-aware and self-loving.

My husband experienced so much pain in his life. He lost his mom at 10 and his father at 18. He threw himself into work to mask the hurt and loss he faced every day. This has turned him into a workaholic who still struggles with expressing his emotions. During the past 20 years I have known him, I have helped teach him how to not just love but be vulnerable and trust others. As with my children, I am my husband's safe space and his home. So no, I am not just a mom. I am not just a wife. I am the G.O.A.T. (Greatest Of All Time) of this shit.

I am someone who constantly kicks fear's ass to the side and goes for it! There are times I fail and times that shit works in my favor. That is life. Not every day and everything will be perfect all the time. There is no one more qualified to show you how to fight through life than a person who does so daily and has become the best version of themselves through not giving up.

Journal Prompt #21: Are you a parent? If so, how does being a parent impact or change your goals? If not, how did your parents influence your life choices?

AFFIRMATIONS:

☐ I belong in important spaces.
☐ I am a good parent.

Reflection

No matter how many times you get knocked down, get up and decide to try again. Take a step back and see what you could have done better or differently. Acknowledge your weaknesses in the situation, work on them, learn from them, and turn them into strengths. You also have to accept that some things may have been out of your control. That is a part of life.

Growing up, in my grandmother's kitchen was the "Serenity Prayer:"

> *God grant me the serenity to accept the things I cannot change, courage to change the things I can, and the wisdom to know the difference.*

This prayer lives with me in my heart. Even if you are not a religious person, you can apply it to your life. While we cannot control the families we are born into, we can create our own. We cannot control how others treat us, but we can control their access to us. We cannot control who loves us, but we can give our love to the ones we decide to. We cannot control that one day we will die, but we can control the life we live.

Journal Prompt #22: What are some things in your life that you have a difficult time accepting you cannot change?

Journal Prompt #23: List things in your life that can change and must, but you have not had the courage to do so yet.

_____

_____

_____

_____

_____

_____

_____

_____

_____

_____

_____

_____

_____

_____

No one knows what is best for you but you. Everybody you know will want to tell you what you should do and who you should be. It may be your mother, your man, or your friends, but you know what they say about opinions and assholes. Everybody has one. But none of those opinions matter if they contradict the body, the career, the marriage, the dreams, the life that you want for yourself. Your husband could love your thick thighs, but you do not. Someone could have told you all your life that you should be a lawyer, an accountant, or a doctor, but you would rather open a boutique or be an artist. You could be the best employee on the team at work, but you hate that damn job and dread going to the office every day.

This is your life. You get to decide what you want to do with it. You get to live for *you*. If you have been seeking approval in your life, today is the day that you stop it. You do not need 5,000 people to approve anything you do. The only person whose approval truly matters is yours. Now is the time to think about what it is that you need to do for yourself to make you happy. Many of us don't even know what it is that will truly make us happy. Material things and accolades often give us a fleeting/temporary feeling of joy, but that kind of happiness isn't what I want you to find. I want you to find your real authentic joy in life. Trust in yourself and believe that you deserve that joy.

Journal Prompt #24: List some things that you need to do in order for you to truly be happy.

_____

_____

_____

_____

_____

_____

_____

_____

_____

_____

_____

_____

_____

_____

As a child, I am sure many people would have described me as being bossy, talkative, and that I thought highly of myself. In reality, especially when I see the reflection of my childhood self through my children, I am not *bossy*. I am a *boss*. I knew my path, and I could easily learn to navigate new challenges. Yes, I was and still am talkative, but those qualities have turned me into who I am today. I have made a career out of asking questions and having an opinion.

To those who said, "She thinks she's all that," well yeah, you were right. I did think so and so should you about yourself. I envy the young girl I once was who was confident and a fearless leader. Now that I am over 30, I am desperately trying to be more like she was. That fierceness was a gift, and if you can carry that into adulthood or learn to ignite it once again, you can have the confidence to conquer your goals.

I was not "all of that" because of how I looked or what I had. I was a little funny-looking, and designer brands outside of Nike did not exist in my world. I was "all that" because I was confident in myself. I loved myself and how well I knew my passions. I liked that other people knew it too. They looked at me with either respect or envy, but no one saw a lost soul who struggled to find herself. Just as I knew and still know who I am deep within, you likely know yourself in the same way. You have to find that inner child and allow them to resurface.

It is time to start being honest with yourself. Time to peel back all the layers of self-doubt and find that confident, bad bitch who is waiting underneath. She is dying to get out. Self-reflection is necessary to know who you are. I like to call myself check-ins. I go over situations that I feel I may not have handled well and ask myself, "How could I have handled something better?"

Journal Prompt #25: Take some time to check in with yourself. How have you been feeling lately? How have you been wanting to feel?

Journal Prompt #26: Are there recent situations in your life where you have done or said something that you regretted or didn't mean? Have you been taking full advantage of every chance you've gotten? If you could go back, how would you have handled yourself and the situation differently?

Journal Prompt #27: Were you a confident child? Are you still confident or have you gained confidence as you've aged? Why or why not?

Journal Prompt #28: Write a letter to your younger self about your childhood dreams and goals. Tell yourself everything you wish you could have known. Tell yourself how you have or plan to take steps to resurface your inner child.

AFFIRMATIONS:

- [ ] Things that I deserve will come to me.
- [ ] I am goal-oriented.
- [ ] My work adds value to the world.
- [ ] I work hard to meet my goals.

The First Step to Change is to Become Aware of Your Own Bullshit

It is time to do the work. Time to uncover the issues that have led you to this point in your life of being frustrated and lacking fulfillment. Facing these issues will help you connect the dots between your past and present. Shit has happened to all of us that was completely out of our control, but there have also been some circumstances that we have created in our lives that made our journeys a little harder. The fact is our lives are a result of both those uncontrollable circumstances and our own choices.

Somewhere around the age of 5 many of us started to gain a sense of self. A lot of that sense of self stems from how others treated us as well as what others told us we were. Much of our lives have been shaped by what other people thought we should do and who they thought we should be. As a child, you are supposed to get good grades in school. At 18, you are supposed to go to college and then get a good job. Eventually, you will buy a house, a car, and have a 700-something credit score. As women, *we* are supposed to find a good man, get married, and have children. As mothers, *we* are expected to raise perfect children regardless of our well-being. As someone who checked many of those boxes all before my 25th birthday, how is it that I was still so unhappy? If I did all that I was told I was supposed to do then should I not be living the dream?

For you, maybe you have a good job. It pays the bills and comes with a nice title to tell people that you have, but it makes you miserable. You are a great mom and you love your kids to the ends of the earth, but you cannot remember the last time you got dressed up for a night out with just your friends, much less went to the bathroom or washed your ass in peace. Maybe you have dreamed about starting a business, but you put your plans on the back burner until the kids were in school. Your youngest is now 10, and your dreams are still sitting there waiting on you. Some of the checklist boxes worked for me, and I am sure some may work for you too. But some of that shit has no alignment with the type of life I wanted, and you may want, to live.

Journal Prompt #29: What are some expectations that others have placed on you? Have you exceeded those expectations yet still remain unhappy?

You are not unhappy because you do not want the life you have. You are not happy because you need more out of life for yourself. Instead of the life that you are living for everybody else, you have to choose to live for yourself. The hard truth is you feel fucking lost because you are following someone else's GPS. Too often we do not want to disappoint others so in return we disappoint ourselves.

Here's the first newsflash: The life you want is on the other side of everybody else's opinions about who you are and what you should be.

One of the biggest lessons of adulthood is that we have to unlearn what others have told us to finally feel fulfilled. That means letting go of your fear of disappointing your family and friends because you do not meet their expectations. You are not the problem, their standards are. What happens if you do not want to go to college, or you never want to get married or have children? Perhaps you are like me and an office job just is not your thing. Then what? Is there no happily-ever-after for us? Where are the speeches about making sure that we are mentally mature, healthy, and happy? We must re-educate ourselves on what it means to live a full life.

I once read a quote from John Lennon that said, *"When I went to school they asked me what I wanted to be when I grew up. I wrote down, happy! They told me that I didn't understand the assignment. And I told them that they didn't understand life."* This quote is one that I use often in my professional and personal life. Checking all the boxes may look great on paper, but who gives a flying fuck what a paper says if you are miserable in real life. Though it does not always feel like it, there is more to life than bills and bullshit. This stops now! It is time for you to stop living for everyone else and do the shit that you want to do to have the life that you want to have.

First, you have to clear out everything that is keeping you from having it. The inner work is the hardest work. You have to face the parts of yourself that you've buried deep. Those are the parts you need to dig deep into. Those are your WHYs. *Why am I the way that I am? Why does this make me shut down or revert back? Why does this trigger me, while that does not?* The answer to all of those things lies in your past, as cliche as it sounds.

While on this journey to self-rediscovery I want you to remember that you are not obligated to be the person you were five years ago, five months ago, or even five minutes ago. Many of us constantly think of the shoulda's, coulda's, and woulda's in our lives, but the truth is we can never go back. We can never change what has already happened. Although our past has shaped us into who we are today, the good and the bad, the past does not define us. We can only work on improving ourselves today, and that involves examining our daily diet. It is not just what we are eating and drinking but everything that we consume. From the TV we watch, the music we listen to, the conversation we participate in, social media, and the people who we surround ourselves with. You are what you eat. So if your life is feeling shitty or is not producing what you want, it is because your daily diet is garbage. Those shitty conversations, people, and toxic social media pages are a huge part of what is holding you back. Negativity almost always outweighs the positive parts of our lives and weighs us down. For me, I physically get pains in my neck and back and cannot sleep when I am consumed with negative feelings or negative energy from others.

Journal Prompt #30: List parts of your current self that you would like to keep with you moving forward. Then, list parts of your current self you would like to leave behind.

Journal Prompt #31: How do your negative feelings manifest physically? How may recognizing and healing the pain that causes those feelings to allow you to feel better physically?

_____

_____

_____

_____

_____

_____

_____

_____

_____

_____

_____

_____

_____

_____

AFFIRMATIONS:

- ☐ My healing is a journey, not a race.
- ☐ I am willing to do the hard work.

Be Proud of Who You Are Instead of Ashamed of Who You Aren't.

WHAT IF WE ALL HAD TO WALK AROUND WITH OUR FAULTS and flaws branded on us like the scarlet letter? Is that who we are? No. We are not our failures. Our flaws do not define who we are. It is how we respond and use those failures that truly define who we are.

Are you really the person who you POST to be on social media? In the digital age, we are all putting our best face forward. We're trying to have the perfect aesthetic, great content, flawless algorithms, filters to make us look 10x better, deep captions from shallow souls. And some people are just being completely fake and phony AF. We are often so consumed with how we appear to others that we've forgotten who we really are. Many of us are allowing the internet to control how we feel. Social media tells us we need to appear and act a certain way in order to be happy or successful, but that's just not true.

Journal Prompt #32: What's your moral compass?

Journal Prompt #33: Who are you when you are alone when no one's watching? Not who you are when you are performing for others.

_____

_____

_____

_____

_____

_____

_____

_____

_____

_____

_____

_____

_____

Journal Prompt #34: What do you do for those who can never repay you?

One of the things that I know and love deeply about myself is that I am me, always. I'm not code-switching for anyone. Some people love it, while some people hate it. All will have to deal.

> *"I walk in every room as myself. I don't walk in any room like anyone else. I'm not cowering. I'm not speaking softly. My voice doesn't change — it sounds exactly the same way. I'm walking as myself and proud..."*
> — Jay Z

Imagine if Puff Daddy, Mary J. Blige, or even Cardi B had changed who they were because they were deemed too ghetto, too urban. Lady Gaga or Dennis Rodman for being too weird. Kate Moss too short. Model Chrissy Teigen and Hollywood royalty Meryl Streep were both told they were too ugly. What if they all had changed because they were told to? They would have lost the qualities that make them uniquely who they are in favor of something more bland and mainstream. You only get to be you in this lifetime. Why be anyone else when you could be yourself?

I want you to spend time with each of these questions and answer them honestly.

Journal Prompt #35: What do you admire the most about yourself?

_____

_____

_____

_____

_____

_____

_____

_____

_____

_____

_____

_____

Journal Prompt #36: What are your biggest strengths?

_____

_____

_____

_____

_____

_____

_____

_____

_____

_____

_____

_____

_____

_____

_____

Journal Prompt #37: What are your biggest weaknesses?

Journal Prompt #38: What's the first thing you do when you wake up in the morning?

Journal Prompt #39: Describe a typical day for you.

Journal Prompt #40: What are you doing often that you love? What are you doing often that you hate?

Journal Prompt #41: Who are the people that you talk to/text or hang out with the most?

Journal Prompt #42: What are you talking about often? How do you feel after those conversations?

Journal Prompt #43: What music are you listening to? What shows are you watching? What social media pages do you frequent?

Journal Prompt #44: At the end of the day, do you typically feel fulfilled or like a failure??

Journal Prompt #45: What daily steps are you taking toward your dream life?

Journal Prompt #46: What are the moments in your life that have shaped you the most?

DO THAT SH!T

Journal Prompt #47: Name 10 adjectives to describe yourself. Design: number to 10

_____

_____

_____

_____

_____

_____

_____

_____

_____

_____

_____

_____

Journal Prompt #48: Now ask two or three people who you feel are the closest to you to give you 10 adjectives to describe you as well. Does anything overlap?

1. _____

2. _____

3. _____

4. _____

5. _____

6. _____

7. _____

8. _____

9. _____

10. _____

DO THAT SH!T

Last question, and I want you to dig deep with this one:

Journal Prompt #49: Who were you before the world told you who to be? That is who the fuck you are and how you find your purpose!

Heal That Shit

"The grass is greener on the other side." No! Some grass is greener because it is fake! My grass is greener because I take care of my damn grass.

— Me, Ashley Brittney Silva

No one: —
   Every therapist ever: "So, tell me about your childhood."

I used to think it was so cliche for therapists, counselors, or psychologists to ask about your childhood. If you are having issues getting along with your coworker Jill at 34, what the flying fuck does that have to do with your childhood? Actually, a lot. The way we are raised, the things we learn or do not learn, and the way we are loved and see love as a child helps mold us into how we love when we are older. The way we are taught to problem-solve as kids usually rears its head as an adult.

"People raised on love see things differently than those raised on survival."

— Joy Marino

Journal Prompt #50: Were you a child who was able to speak freely about your feelings, or were you told to shut up and act a certain way?

___
___
___
___
___
___
___
___
___
___
___
___
___
___

Journal Prompt #51: Were you a child who was given things in abundance without having to do anything for them, or were you only rewarded when you got good grades or behaved well? How has that shaped you?

DO THAT SH!T

Whenever I ask my mom why she felt like our relationship turned poorly when I was younger, she simply says, "Because you were bad." My mother would also jokingly call me Rhoda. She was the main character in the 1956 film *The Bad Seed*. She was a cute 8-year-old with pigtails. She was also a murderer.

/bad/
Adjective
1. Of poor quality or low standard
2. Not such as to be hoped for or desired; unpleasant or unwelcome

Journal Prompt #52: Are there things your parents or other influential people in your life said to you as a child that have stuck with you to this day? Things that impacted your confidence or the way you see yourself?

My grandmother called me "Cakes" because I was a chubby kid. She had me sit at the kitchen table and pinch my nose for several minutes every day because it was too wide. My grandmother would also emphasize to us as children not to spend too much time in the summer sun, or we would get too dark.

I stopped eating eggs at about 6. I had heard talk about how egg yolks cause high cholesterol and make you gain weight, so no eggs for me. I also chose to stop eating pork and beef around 10 so that I wouldn't gain much weight.

I am still very self-conscious about my weight and my nose. My mother and sister have always been thin. My sister can eat like a full high school football team and not gain a pound. If I look at a piece of cake too hard, I gain five pounds. I've always been a curvier girl carrying most of my weight in my legs. I have times when I go extremely hard in the gym and go on strict diets if the scale goes over my "fat" weight. My depression will kick into high gear if the scale tips that number. I have toyed with the idea of getting a nose job since I was 14 years old. Maybe one day I will. It is something that I am still insecure about, and if and when I decide to do it, it's my face. No one else's. Insecurities are a part of life. We all have them. I love my complexion, but there are those moments on vacation where I think, "OK, maybe you've had enough sun."

One Valentine's Day, my grandmother gave my sister and me both mugs with candy inside. My sister's mug was cute, white with red hearts that said I LOVE YOU very large. My mug was hideous. I hated it! It was purposely dented and read: I LOVE YOU with all your "im perfeck shuns." My "im perfeck shuns" is a roundabout way to say imperfections, but I was around 10 years old and had no idea what a pun was or how to interpret a metaphor. While writing this, I looked up the mug online and found it. Wow. Exactly how I remember it. I still hate it! That mug became the way I defined myself. I was bad, fucked up, dented, ugly, not good enough, and misunderstood—a sentiment that I carried well into my adult life.

My sister was what some might consider the perfect child. She was pretty, sweet, and innocent. She did not talk a lot, and she did not talk back. When I came along, I was the exact opposite. I have been affectionately called *Mouth Almighty* because I talked too much. I questioned everything, and I had an answer for everything. The complete opposite of what most adults, especially old-school adults, like or consider good in a child.

I was not blind to the fact that my sister was my grandmother's favorite. As a child, I never felt like anyone's favorite. Well there was one person, Johnny. Johnny was my grandmother's boyfriend, who I considered my grandfather. Johnny always made me feel so special, safe, and loved. Johnny would drive me to school each morning while the rest of my friends walked. One day, I decided I wanted to start walking to school with my friends and he let me. Unbeknownst to me, every day as I walked to school Johnny followed closely behind. He passed away when I was only about 7, but I think of him often, and I know how much he loved and cared for me. At times when I am feeling alone, I often get a calming sensation over me that I feel to be him.

At school, I had my set of friends but unbeknownst to my family, some girls picked on me daily. I hid the fact that this was happening with pseudo-confidence. I pretended that I was fine and that I felt so confident with myself, but I wasn't. I still felt dented and unworthy. In middle school, the meanness from girls got worse until one day I decided to fight back and never stopped. From that moment on I knew that I had always to defend myself whether it was with my words or my fists. Never again would I let anyone think that they could hurt me, physically or emotionally.

I always felt sad, overlooked, and guarded. This hardness turned me into what some may call a bitch. I knew others interpreted my honesty and mood as being a bitch. Because of that, I played the role more often than not. So many times in my life I have been straight-up bitchy or mean to people I didn't know. Some I had just met, and even those that I have known forever. Sometimes it was because I was having a fucked-up day. Other times it was because I was feeling shitty about my life or feeling insecure about what I had conjured up in my head that people thought of me. I began to assume the worst in others, and I would lash out at anyone I felt was attacking, judging, or hurting me. The way I reacted out of fear took a lot of unlearning. I have learned to take accountability for the way I have shown up when I wasn't at my best, which includes learning to apologize when I take out my anger or hurt on someone else who does not deserve it.

Journal Prompt #53: Have you ever had any unhealthy defense mechanisms that you've unlearned or still need to unlearn?

DO THAT SH!T

I launched my first website, IAMSUPERGORGE.com (IASG) when I was 25. It lasted for a little over five years. The site was my baby. I put my everything into it, working night and day on it. Along with the website, we also had an accompanying online radio show. I just knew that IASG was my IT. It was going to lead me to work for a large entertainment news station like BET or E! and all of my dreams would come true. But every time I experienced a high with IASG, I had months upon months of very low lows. No interviews, no paid gigs, nothing but 24-hour days of work day after day. At this time, a peer who had started her blog around the same time as I had left our area and moved to LA. Her career then seemingly flourished with hosting jobs and multiple TV appearances while I was at a complete halt. I was upset, and I was jealous. Why not me?

Finally, I got tired of fighting for a dream that I wasn't even sure I was still meant to have. I got so angry with myself for spending all this time and money on a "fantasy dream" that I decided maybe I wasn't supposed to be happy or successful in a career. Maybe I was supposed to just be a wife and a mom. Maybe God put me on this earth to only focus on nurturing my kids, supporting my husband, and being there for my family and friends. If he wanted me to be happy, it would have happened by now, right?

I threw every bit of energy I had into my family. Cooking and cleaning constantly. Making sure my kids were in every activity they wanted to be in. Running myself into exhaustion so that they were everywhere on time even when they had activities in different parts of town at the same time. I made sure I showed up for every event anyone in my life had even when I was dead tired or had to spend money I didn't have on a sitter. I made sure my husband always felt supported in his endeavors. I would ask my children after every outing or gift I had gotten them if they liked it and if they were happy. Because I wasn't happy and if I wasn't, I needed reassurance that at least my children were. I felt this massive pressure to overachieve as a wife and a mom. My husband worked 16-hour days multiple days of the week. I would often attend weddings and family functions alone. Our date nights were months and months apart. My friends would plan couples' trips or double-date nights, and I wouldn't be invited because they knew my husband would have to work. I had remained supportive of his career and tried not to complain, but the truth was I felt like a single-married mom. Married on paper but alone all the time in real life.

In the pits of my soul, I was angry with God. Why would He give me such huge dreams, talents, and goals, only for me not to achieve them? I recall a day screaming to the top of my lungs at God. Maybe if I cried hard enough and yelled hard enough, He would hear me this time and answer my prayers. But nothing changed. Well, one thing did–my belief in myself. It was completely gone.

The days during that time became a run-on blurry sentence. One blank feeling after another. I no longer looked forward to what was in store for me. My days consisted of being a good wife, lonely as hell, making sure the kids were to school on time, getting good grades, and keeping up with if it was my week to be my kids' sports team snack bitch. I was pouring everything that I had into my kids, my husband, and those around me to make sure that they knew how much I loved them, but eventually, I was pouring from an empty cup. I had given my all to everyone around me, leaving nothing for myself.

The ending of my blog came after I went back and forth about an interview request with a well-known celebrity. Everything was going great, There was a date and time set. This was going to be the big break that my blog needed. Once the big day was approaching the emails from the celebrity's publicist abruptly stopped. I emailed and emailed with no response. Finally, I gave up. I remember feeling so defeated and thought this was the sign just to let go of my dream. I started to cry there on my living room floor in front of the couch, and then the crying turned into sobbing. The crying, sobbing, and gasping for air lasted for almost 24 hours. In those hours, I felt that everything I ever wanted, career-wise, was gone.

The next morning, my husband and I just so happened to have a doctor's appointment with our new primary doctor. When we arrived, I wore dark sunglasses. My face was swollen, and my eyes were bloodshot red from all the crying. When the doctor walked in, she immediately asked my husband to step out of the room. She asked me if I was ok. I said yes, I was just having a bad day. And then the tears and sobbing started. By the end of my appointment, I was diagnosed with severe clinical depression and given a referral to a psychiatrist.

After I was officially diagnosed with depression, I felt a sense of relief. Like a weight was finally lifted off of my shoulders. All the sad and cloudy days, all the days not being able to get out of bed, all the days and nights that I couldn't sleep, all of the constant body pains, the overthinking, the constant doubt, I finally knew the reason for them. Despite my relief, I didn't truly want to face my ailment. I was afraid of how other people would judge me. Depression was still so taboo in the Black community. It's too common for Black women to hide their struggles because it is embedded in our character to be "strong Black women" who carry the world on our backs without complaints. It's damaging. Those close to me who I did decide to tell, I shared with them the diagnosis but sugar-coated it. I told them that I had lingering post-partum depression. My youngest was a little over one at the time, and I felt that post-partum would be more acceptable to say. People are usually more sympathetic to pregnant women or to those who just had a baby.

Journal Prompt #54: Do you battle with mental illness? How did you discover that mental illness, and how did you feel when diagnosed?

But the truth was, I had known that something had been wrong with me for years. I knew I had been depressed for over a decade. Going back to my teenage years, I felt the switch when I stopped being happy and my lust for life started to fade. There was nothing that gave me that joyous feeling that I was so desperately wanting. I had always been ashamed to seek help. I was afraid of the stigma. Afraid because I had been told that I didn't have anything to be depressed about and that I didn't look depressed. Other people had much less or way worse situations than I did, so I should shut up and be grateful.

Let me explain. Depression does not discriminate. It does not care about your age, your race, your gender, or if you live in a mansion or a shelter. It doesn't care about your marital status, and it doesn't care what your bank account says. Depression can affect you regardless of how others view your "perfect" life. While we may not all suffer from mental illness, all of our mental health will be affected at some point in our lives.

I decided that instead of hiding my depression, I would start to talk about it openly, especially on social media. This was years before mental health became a "trending topic." It was scary at first to be so open about it, but I found it easier for me to blindly talk about my depression with strangers on social media versus talking to those closest to me. Many of those who I had decided to open up to about my diagnosis in real life weren't as supportive as I'd have liked them to be.

I was met with comments like, "Why do you need to tell people?" "You have nothing to be depressed about," or "You are in your 20s living a good life with a providing husband."

Once I started with the psychiatrist, she gave me a prescription for antidepressants and a therapist referral sheet. Immediately I filled my prescription and went through the list of psychologists.

The next week I was at a psychologist's office, telling her all about my childhood. The entire time I watched her as she watched the clock, waiting for my 60 minutes to be over.

At the end of the appointment, she said, "Ok, that is it for today. See the front desk and pay your copay. Oh, and make your next appointment."

That was IT! I wasn't healed, and she hadn't helped me with shit! For the next few weeks, I returned with the same outcome. Not until around week four was there progress, finally.

At the end of our session, she said, "Do you think that your mom would accompany you to your next session?"

I said, "I will ask."

When I returned home, I called my mom, and surprisingly, she agreed to go with me to my next appointment. But the next week came and went, and my mom never showed up. There was always some excuse why she couldn't make it. Eventually, I stopped asking. After about two months into therapy, I quit. I also stopped taking my antidepressants because they weren't helping. I still felt shitty all the time. The only thing that they seemed to do was stop my crying. By that I mean my eyes literally weren't producing water.

Over the next five years, life just kept on "life-ing" with bullshit after bullshit. There was a break-in at my home. Luckily, we weren't there at the time, but all of my expensive items were stolen. I no longer felt safe in the house that we'd worked so hard to get and that we were raising our two children in. I stopped trusting some of the people who were around me, including the consistent babysitter we'd finally found. After the break-in, I was unable to sleep and developed insomnia. For the next five years, I maybe averaged two hours of sleep a night. Eventually, when we decided to move, the few weeks leading up to the move were very hard on me. I gained 30 pounds in less than four weeks. I was working out daily, but the weight was piling on. Not only had I fallen deeper into depression, but I was suffering from anxiety and PTSD.

The break-in put a strain on my entire life. I tried a new therapist with no luck. I even chose one named Janet Jackson because, well, I love Janet Jackson. Over the next few years, my marriage was less than stellar. I was in a deep, dark hole of sadness all the time, and my husband didn't understand why I couldn't just snap out of it. He would often say that he didn't understand why being a wife and a mom wasn't enough for me. We'd argue and fuss a lot. I felt like I was in a one-sided marriage that was just never going to get better. My husband felt he was married to someone who complained all the time, and we both wanted out of the miserable routine.

Soon after, my mother was diagnosed with Stage 4 lymphoma cancer. This diagnosis was tough, but in my heart of hearts, I knew she was going to beat it. And she did. But only three months after going into remission, her cancer was back and more aggressive. The chemotherapy wasn't working. She was going to need a stem cell transplant and a minimum of a month's stay in the hospital. My sister and I were both tested to be stem cell donors. I wasn't a match, but luckily my sister was. Not being a match again made me feel like I was a failure to my mother. I couldn't save her. The stem cell transplant was a success, but her months-long stay in the hospital was anything but easy. She lost more weight and was sick all the time. One day while visiting my mom, we sat and talked. I had to leave to make my hour-and-a-half drive back home to get my daughter to dance practice. I got home, got my daughter dressed for dance, and was about to head out the door when I noticed that I had a missed call from the hospital.

"Mrs. Silva, your mother has become unresponsive, and you should get to the hospital immediately."

I sped back, calling my sister, husband, godsisters, and best friend on the way to meet me there. When we arrived, my mother looked frailer than she had just hours earlier. She was hooked up to a breathing machine. It felt like this could be the end.

Journal Prompt #55: Have you ever experienced a big loss or event that changed the course of your life? How did that impact the way you saw or treated yourself?

After my mom was released, she still had almost daily doctor visits. I had to make the hour-plus drive to and from the visits. When my sister or I were unable to make it, I would order Ubers for mom back and forth home. I was trying to be there for my mom physically and emotionally as much as possible, but I was also dealing with all of this too. If you've ever been a caregiver for someone who is battling a potentially fatal illness, then you know that it takes a huge toll on you. I never showed my pain to anyone except for my husband, and when I did, instead of him consoling me, he broke down crying. A man I had only seen cry maybe twice in the almost 20 years of knowing him. His mother and stepmother had both died from cancer, and now he felt like he was losing his mother-in-law to the disease. So I did what I always did, I put my feelings to the side and consoled him. Inside I was furious. This was the time I needed him, someone, anyone to be there for me, and I felt completely alone and unable to put my armor down. So I drank, drank, and drank some more, all the while increasingly becoming more depressed and angrier.

As a positive outlet, I threw myself into work for my podcast. Planning, producing, editing, etc., but my podcast wasn't growing. Our viewership was much lower than I had anticipated. All this hard work, again, wasn't paying off. Over a few months, my friendships started to fall off as well. I didn't feel as though many of my friends were there for me in the capacity that I needed them to be, and it made me bitter toward them. My mother would berate me on the days I couldn't physically be there for her and take her to appointments, and my marital issues were still occurring. For the millionth time in my life, I felt like a failure. No matter how hard I tried and worked, I was constantly failing and constantly hurting. Finally, it all felt like too much for me to continue to try and handle. There never seemed to be any glimmer of hope for me or my life. I wanted it all to end. So, that is what I tried to do. I tried to take my own life.

Journal Prompt #56: At your darkest moments, how did you feel? What kept you going?

I do not want to get into the details of what happened because it is something that I am still healing from and probably will be for years to come. As I am still healing from the repressed childhood trauma of an older cousin of my stepsisters laying beside me and asking me if I was going to be a virgin forever at 8 while he was babysitting us or being drugged by a guy in my teens and blacking out. These are things that have wounded me. Things that are deep and personal that I am actively healing from. Experiences that I thought I'd "gotten over," but I'd simply pushed them far to the back of my mind and never did the work to properly heal.

So I had to turn my mind away from my family, my friends, and my business and turn it on myself. I was fucked up, and the only person who could help me was me. So that is what I did at the hospital after a suicide attempt. They asked me if I wanted to stay, and I wanted to tell them "no" so badly. I wanted to do what I normally would do, what came naturally, and that was to tell them that nothing was wrong with me. That I was just having another bad day. The truth was, I was not having a bad day or a bad week, or even a bad month. I was having a bad life. And as much as I tried to pray or wish things would change, they hadn't. I knew that I needed to seek professional help, as I had done before, but this time I had to take it seriously. I could not give up on my healing and treatment because it didn't work as fast as the timeline I'd set. So I decided not to say that I was OK. I wasn't. I needed immediate help, and if I would have gone home, I would've returned feeling just as bad as I did when I arrived.

A week-long hospital stay later and once released, I didn't magically feel better. I felt just as shitty as the day I went in, if not worse. My sister picked me up from the hospital instead of my husband. He felt that I was selfish for trying to take my own life, which is a statement that I often hear people say when referring to those who are suicidal or have died by suicide. Selfish? SELFISH? Imagine all the dark days this person has lived through for others, not for themselves, so that they wouldn't be deemed selfish. He had no idea of my daily thoughts. I was constantly secretly wishing for death so the pain would end.

When I returned home from the hospital, the house was empty. My kids were at school, and my husband was not there to greet me. My wallet was sitting on the kitchen counter. My credit card and bank card had all been taken out because they were in my husband's name. Another painful blow. I knew at that moment I would never let my husband, or anyone else for that matter, have financial power over me again.

I immediately returned to my normal way of life, Two days after I checked out of the hospital, I hosted an event with a huge smile on my face. Over the next few weeks, I celebrated multiple friends' birthdays. None knew what I was dealing with. I was still suffering, still feeling overwhelmed, and still full of sadness. Even more so that I couldn't open up emotionally to anyone. What I needed was support and to work through my struggles.

About a year later, after consistently taking my antidepressants, going to therapy, getting back into a routine of working out, and finally losing the 30 pounds I had gained years ago, my husband and I were in a good place. I had made new friends, and I felt like I had found a new lease on life. And then life hit me with two major blows back to back.

If you've experienced cancer or have been a care provider for someone who has had cancer, you know that even when the cancer is "gone," it's not. It's simply gone "today." Every three months the survivor has to be tested to make sure the cancer is still at bay. One day, my mom was waiting for her three-month test results. Each time this happens, I hold my breath a little longer, and my heart seems to beat faster and slower simultaneously. That night I decided to go out for dinner and drink with two of my girlfriends to relieve some stress. Dinner was great. The drinks were better. Leaving dinner, it started to snow unexpectedly. So I decided I needed to rush home before the roads got bad. As I left the restaurant, I was pulled over for going slightly over the white line at a red light. I'd been asked if I had been drinking. I had. More than the legal limit. I was taken to a police station and charged with a DUI. Ten minutes later, I was headed home. I was upset. I was embarrassed. I had been drinking. I legally was over the limit. But drunk I wasn't. But that's no excuse. I broke the law as too many of us have done. Lesson learned.

A few weeks later, I learned that I was unexpectedly pregnant and soon suffered a painful miscarriage that I never talked to anyone about besides my husband. We weren't trying for another baby. We both have been very clear that we are happy having two children, but alongside the physical pain came unexpected grief. How could I be grieving for a child that I didn't want? Was God punishing me for having an abortion at 18? Or was I finally releasing all the tears and pain that had been built up over the past few years from my marriage, the break-in, my career, my mom's diagnosis, and losing friends? I felt so confused. I decided not to tell anyone, but holding it in only made me lash out more at the people closest to me. I was tired of being a constant "Look at how sad I am" party of one.

By this point in my life, I turned into someone who downplayed things that had happened to me–including significant things like my mom's cancer battle. Some of my friends' parents have passed away. How dare I talk to them about my sadness and my mom being in the hospital with cancer when their parents are gone? My suicide attempt and hospital stay were secrets to everyone aside from my husband, best friend, and sister. No one else in my life at the time knew. I tried to tell others, but it seemed like the time was never right or that they didn't care.

Regarding my miscarriage, I knew people who had suffered miscarriages and even had children stillborn who wanted those children, so I felt it was selfish for me to grieve a child I didn't want. But I was grieving. Not only had my body gone through a traumatic experience but my mental state, which I had been working heavily on, was affected. All my hard work for myself seemed to be undone in a blink.

A little over a week later, it was a friend's birthday, and I should have stayed home. Physically I was ok, but emotionally I was a wreck. Regardless of how I felt, I showed up. That's who I am. Birthdays are important. When I arrived for lunch, it turned out to be a double date, and I realized I wasn't technically invited. This wasn't communicated to me, and I felt left out. Not being included is a huge emotional trigger for me. I should have left, but I had just taken an hour Uber ride, and I was hungry. I got extremely drunk and had a complete meltdown. Tears. Cussing. Fussing. Still, I told no one about the miscarriage. Again I felt how selfish it would be to say at that moment "Happy Birthday. I had a miscarriage last week. Let's celebrate." Instead, I just cried, argued, and embarrassed myself. Afterward, that friendship faded out. I never told her what was going on with me at the time.

Journal Prompt #57: Have you ever started healing and had a major setback? What was that like and how did you overcome it?

Journal Prompt #58: Over the years, how have your friendships changed as you've changed?

Journal Prompt #59: Have you ever felt like you had to keep your emotions a secret from the outside world? Has that secrecy impacted your healing journey?

AFFIRMATIONS:

- ☐ I deserve to be heard.
- ☐ My feelings are not selfish. They are not burdens.
- ☐ It is OK not to be OK.

Realization

MY GRANDMOTHER WAS BORN IN THE 1930s IN THE SOUTH. She experienced racism and grew up during the brown paper bag era. Our Black features, such as a big nose like mine, weren't the standard of beauty. So the things that my grandmother said to me about my weight, complexion, or nose weren't out of a place of malice. It was simply the way she was raised and knew life.

My sister was a sweet child, mild-mannered, and didn't talk back. Then I came along, and I was the exact opposite. I talked too much; took my sister's things, including her clothes; and lost her high school ring. I wasn't a terrible child, I was just a little sister. A little sister who, like most younger siblings, was the troublemaker or the one who just might need a bit more attention.

I wasn't a perfect child, but I wasn't bad. I am not a bad seed or a rotten fruit. I am me, and I deserve to be loved, even with all my "Imprefeckshuns."

I have learned that some people do not mean to be rude, hurtful, mean, unsupportive, etc., myself included. They probably aren't aware of the harm they are causing or recognize why they are causing it. That takes self-discovery and accountability. That takes seeing someone else's life and recognizing their traumatic experiences, or as Oprah likes to ask, "What happened to you?" instead of writing them off as a horrible person.

Maybe my mom didn't know how to support me. Maybe limits were put on her dreams as a child, so in return, she tried to limit mine. Over time, I have come to understand that my mom's flaws were just that. Flaws. She, like the rest of us, is a human being who is learning as she goes. She is adapting and growing. There are times and will be times when she, like the rest of us, comes up short. When I became a mom, I began to understand my mother more and more. How at times, we fall short of reaching that high pedestal society places mothers on. I also see how, though we may fall short, we are responsible for our own flaws and mistakes. When we can grow with those mistakes, then we can begin healing. I cannot go back in time and heal my mother or change what happened. I can begin to heal, not only my inner child but through the lens of being a mother, and my relationship with my mother as well.

Recognizing your flaws and mistakes and healing them is a process we will continue throughout the rest of our lives. I have lashed out and was a mean bitch to others—some because they deserved it, but many didn't. Many got the wrath of me that stemmed from a place of pain and insecurities. A place where I constantly felt judged or looked over. That wasn't fair to them.

Though my husband was not there for me in every way I needed him to be, I started to recognize that there were things in his life that impacted his reaction to my suffering. He didn't understand how I could willingly want to take myself away from him and our children, knowing the impact losing his mother had on him. I had to be empathetic, but that emotion was a hard practice when I felt so unseen.

I cried alone. I wiped my own tears.

> **SUICIDE PREVENTION OUTREACH**
>
> Suicide is never the answer. If you know someone who has tried to commit suicide, do not reprimand them. Do not accuse them of being selfish or state that they were trying to take the easy way out. This is the furthest thing from the truth. Speaking as a suicide survivor, I no longer wanted to live with daily negative thoughts about myself or feel like a burden to the ones I loved. What the hurting person needs the most from you is your support and professional help.

My deepening depression started to get in the way of the one thing I have always felt great at, being a mom. I had become easily irritated with pick-ups, drop-offs, and helping with homework. I would find myself lashing out at my children at times that they didn't deserve it. I wasn't cooking and cleaning the house the way I normally had in the past because I simply didn't feel like it. So I playfully created an alter ego named Ms. Pearly Mae to help me cope with the exhaustion of motherhood. Ms. Pearly Mae is an older, strict, take-no-nonsense woman. A nanny type from Jamaica, although my accent sucks. She was based on the late great Robin Williams character, Mrs. Doubtfire, with a few obvious differences. She created laughs between my children and me during times I wanted to scream or cry.

That alter ego held me together as a mom. Ms. Pearly Mae came out in my hardest moments because when you're a mom, you can't take breaks from it. When I felt that I needed a break or I would break myself, I switched on my alter ego. Slipping into her allowed me to not only parent my kids but heal myself. She guided me back to reality and allowed me to let go of my fears and just be someone else. We all find our coping mechanisms, and some are healthier than others. For me, Ms. Pearly Mae showed me not to take life so seriously. She brought back a bond with my kids that had been breaking, and she showed me that sometimes, laughter is life's best medicine.

Although my husband, who I have known for more than half of my life, wasn't there for me emotionally the way I needed him to be, I've had to forgive him for not loving me properly when he didn't know how. He had to mature mentally, and maturing takes work that sometimes feels near impossible to complete.

Following my attempt to take my own life, those first few weeks after I was home, I started mentally preparing for my divorce. We were both done. My husband didn't deserve nor was he asking for my forgiveness. Our vows were for better or worse. At his worst, I have been there helping him to pick up the pieces. At my worst, he abandoned me. That was the nail in the coffin that showed me how little my life mattered. I didn't see my world having meaning, and I was being proven right by the person who should have been showing me the opposite. No one knew that was going on. I carried on with my life. I kept showing up. I continued on, all while being gutted inside.

Journal Prompt #60: Have you ever felt disappointed by the way someone you care about has treated you? How did that impact the way you viewed them and yourself?

_____

_____

_____

_____

_____

_____

_____

_____

_____

_____

_____

_____

_____

One day something changed between my husband and I.

We started talking again. We vowed to be better spouses, and my husband took accountability for the pain he'd inflicted on me. He took accountability for not living up to his vows. I am a forgiver. I love hard. I love my husband unconditionally. I also had to take accountability for myself. I'd neglected my mental health, my well-being, for far too long. I hid how deeply I was hurt by those closest to me. I was not seeking professional help. That wasn't fair to my husband or any of my family members and friends. I had to stop putting on a facade that everything was ok because it wasn't. I learned to be open and honest with my husband whenever I was down or felt myself sinking into a low place. We started doing check-ins with each other, and slowly, day after day, we began to heal together.

I decided to start addressing things head-on as they happened. Letting them linger only caused more unnecessary frustrations. Bad thoughts, times, and feelings do not need to fester. This has been a huge part of my healing. Those who have not yet healed aren't mentally mature, do not understand the healing process, or are unwilling to heal because they are devoted to misunderstanding just won't get it. That's on them.

Heal for yourself first and then for and with each other.

Hitting rock bottom taught me the most valuable lesson. It taught me to love and put myself first.

My husband is always the center of attention. At a club or party, the DJ is the nucleus. He's used to all eyes being on him and being praised. For the majority of our relationship, I was a constant cheerleader, telling him how much I admired him and how great he was. As I sank deeper into my depression, I stopped doing that. Although not an excuse for him to treat me how I had been treated, he felt that I had abandoned him in a way too by no longer being that cheerleader. What I also realized was I had not only allowed this treatment from him, but I'd taught him to put my feelings on the back burner. I taught him that it was ok to put his work, his dreams, and his life before mine and that I'd still be there cheering.

I do not allow this any longer. For anyone reading this, if you are allowing anyone to make you feel as though you are on the back burner or you are sub-tiered to them, this stops today. You are the main character in your life. Place yourself at the forefront of your life. Not only that, expect those around you to cheer as loudly as you are for yourself. If the people in your life cannot cheer you on, then they do not have your best interests at heart. The people who truly care for you will be your personal team of cheerleaders. Your success is their success and vice versa. They watch you succeed and feel proud. Do not keep people in your life who do not want you to succeed.

The good news is that some of your worst days are behind you. Some of your best days are ahead of you. And you haven't even met everyone who will love and support you yet.

The right people will get you, and the right people will love you.

The right people will see your worth and try to understand and help your battles because we all have them. There are people who will work to be by your side through thick and thin, and there are those who will walk out of your life because you are too difficult. It's a sucky part of life, but it is a part that many of us will experience. People will come and go. People will leave you at your hardest and criticize you at your best. There will always be someone who wants you in their life but will not put in the effort to keep you there.

Sometimes, God has people walk out on you because He knew you would never walk out on them.

We often hold onto or want to hold onto things that we've outgrown. The people who are supporting your progress, being a helping hand when you need it, those people will grow with you. Those who are not, those who do not cheer when you achieve something or surpass them, they are like pots that have become too small for a plant to continue growing. They are not your people.

Not everyone will stick around, and not everyone deserves to. I've had friendship break-ups that have broken my heart more than any ex-boyfriend ever did. But through losing those friendships, I built even stronger ones. I have learned to identify the qualities missing from my ex-friends and identify them in new people. I have found what went wrong in the past and learned from those mistakes so that my new relationships will begin with a strong foundation. I have learned to find people who will not leave me, regardless of the work that has to be done.

There will be people who will quit on you. Don't be one of them.

Fear often impacts the way we treat our relationships. I am slowly letting my armor down to extend grace to those I love, the same way I want grace in return. I've opened up to letting new people in my life and made some of the best friends I have ever had. I had to let go of the notion that I would constantly be let down by others, by my dreams, and by myself. In the past, I have feared others not choosing me, which forced me to choose myself. Now that I have chosen myself, I also have to learn how to choose others by finding those who want to pick me just the same.

One of the greatest gifts in life that we can receive and give is the gift of genuine friendship and support.

Journal Prompt #61: Are you requiring more from others than you give? Are you giving more than you're getting or the other way around? How does this impact you and your relationships?

My hurt, my pain, and my unwillingness to seek help and change were my biggest hindrances. I learned that I had to let all that pain go. It took me three decades of carrying around emotional baggage to do so, but I finally released it. I honestly felt no hatred or ill will toward anyone. I was holding myself prisoner in a jail of sadness, hurt, and depression. I was blocking myself from growth.

I now like to deal with my issues head-on, no matter how big or small they may seem. I do not let them linger. I cannot change anyone else's behavior. I cannot change anything that has happened in my past. I am only in control of myself and my healing, and I have chosen to heal. I have decided to heal for myself, my happiness, my peace, and my future. That is the way that I control the trajectory of my life.

I'll reiterate that things happen to each and every one of us in our lives. We use those things to either be a victim or as our testimony.

Most of us have a lot to unpack and do not even realize it. We are carrying around baggage that is weighing us down.

I stopped self-loathing. I stopped playing my sad story over and over in my head. I stopped blaming everyone else. I stopped posting sad-ass "My life is miserable" memes and quotes I had found on Instagram. If you're doing that too, stop that shit. It is drawing more sadness and misery into your life. The law of attraction is very real.

I wasn't OK. I was broken, frustrated, and felt completely uncertain. I realized that I had to decide to put myself back together. I committed to refocusing on my own healing instead of simply trying to move on with life to no avail like so many people try to do. And the largest part of my healing included compassion and forgiveness for others and myself.

I have evolved as a woman. I do not feel malice. I do not seek revenge. Karma spins the block every time.

"...Life is going to do what it is going to do. And we are all going to get chin-checked by life one way or another. So I might as well focus on my enlightenment and roll with the river and not fight with the rocks."
— Lauren London

Journal Prompt #62: What are some issues you have now that you've been putting off resolving?

Journal Prompt #63: Have you currently or in the past fallen into a pit of self-despair? How did you get out of it, or have you taken steps to get out of it?

Journal Prompt #64: Do you believe in karma? What does karma mean to you?

AFFIRMATIONS:

- ☐ I take accountability for my actions.
- ☐ I have the strength to pull myself out of this.
- ☐ I am the hero of my own story.

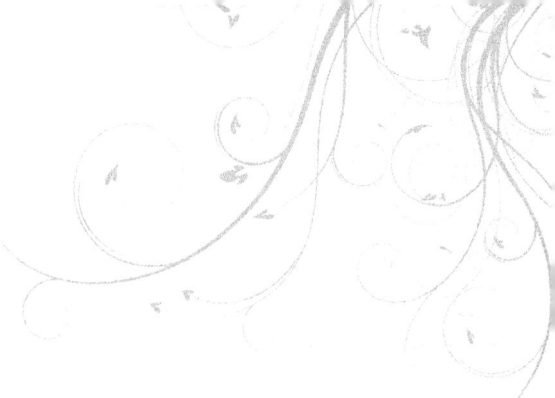

The Work

DO NOT SPEND THE REST OF YOUR LIFE PLAYING THE VICTIM. It is time for a new role.

You do not have to suffer in silence. Throw the notion of "sweeping it under the rug" out of the window.

I recently realized that I held so much in because I had never felt safe sharing my pain or even my joys with those around me. Even though I was constantly surrounded by others, I lacked confidants–individuals who would listen and respect my privacy and hard moments. That is something that I desperately prayed for.

Diminishing my own traumas was one of the ways I thought that I was coping.

Have you ever seen this quote?

> "Never tell your problems to anyone. 80% do not care, and 20% are glad you have them."

That is how I felt. Finding your safe space/circle is extremely important. I have never understood those who proudly say they don't need friends or family. I realize that those people have probably been hurt by others and need to heal.

Certain people have gotten horrible and shitty versions of me because I didn't trust them.

I have cultivated a safe space, my circle, which is small. I used to think I needed a bunch of friends. I thought that I needed many people who liked me. I wanted popularity, but with it comes not having truly close friends. I can know a lot of people, but friends? That word is now only reserved for a select deserving few—those who truly know me and who I know.

Find your safe spaces and friends, those who are happy for you when you succeed, and those who comfort you when you are at your lowest.

Often when you want to address something that has been done to hurt you or harm you, people often perceive that as being difficult or toxic. What they really mean is they'd rather continue living the story that they have created in their own head instead of the story that requires them to own up to or take responsibility for their actions.

Journal Prompt #65: Do you have a circle of close friends or confidants who you can go to in times of trouble? How has that impacted your life?

I decided I didn't want to be surrounded by people who I had to internalize my feelings with. I wanted people around me who I could go to when I was happy as fuck, when I was successful as fuck, and who would be as happy for me and my success. I wanted people around me who would acknowledge and support me through the hard times as well.

Now that I feel like I have finally found a place of mental maturity, I try to use the same thought process on myself as I do when seeking out my close friends. I think daily about if I met my current self, would I want to be my own friend?

Journal Prompt #66: Would you want to be friends with your current self? Why or why not?

Mental maturity also leads us to know that we do not have to respond to everything that upsets us. That was a hard one for me to grasp, as I am expressive. I once read, "There are two types of pain. One that hurts you, and the other that changes you."

It is not fair to others to act out or say, "It is just the way I am." People are not mind readers.

"You just do not understand."

You are right. They do not. How can someone understand if you do not talk to them and if you do not express your feelings?

Learn to be patient and give grace to others. You could be dealing with something that they know nothing about, and they could be too. We are all human, and we are all flawed.

We often think of putting ourselves first as selfish, especially as women. We put our kids first, our spouse, our parents, friends, and even work. That is not helpful. It is not helpful to them, and it is definitely not helpful to you. You cannot pour from an empty glass. I have tried, and it didn't work. I was miserable when I was in the deepest, darkest place of my depression, and my entire household suffered. No clothes were being washed, no food was getting cooked, and no fun was being had. My husband would often tell me how much my depression was affecting our marriage. I knew it was, but what I had a really hard time with was that he couldn't see that as much as it was affecting the kids and our marriage, It was 10 times worse for me. I was suffering, and I needed to take responsibility for my recovery. If no one recognized my needs, I would need to tend to them myself. The first step of healing is to recognize that you need to heal and in order to do that, you have to be willing to put in the work. Your healing, real healing, is your responsibility. Only you can do that.

I let myself feel those human emotions because they are real. I have to work through them, not just get over them. I have to acknowledge the source and realize my triggers to connect the dots.

Journal Prompt #67: Allow yourself to feel how you are feeling right now. Write down the things that have been troubling you and the things that have been lightening your spirit.

Communication, having simple conversations, is the most mature thing that I believe anyone can do. We are humans who often do not interpret things as they are. We let others influence our narratives or shape events that could be handled with a simple conversation.

We cannot heal, we cannot grow, and we won't evolve while holding on to what has hurt us. Let that shit go.

What are you doing for your mental health to heal? I am a true believer in prayer, but sometimes you do need more than prayer. No matter what your momma, your grandma, your pastor, or anyone else tells you, everything cannot simply be prayed away. If that were the case, most of us would be living the lives of our dreams all the time. Seeking therapy does not mean that you are "crazy." You need to speak to someone with an unbiased opinion who does not know you from Adam and Eve. Someone who is trained to give you the proper tools to heal yourself. We have to start taking our mental health as seriously as we do the things that attack our physical bodies. Why is it that we are in such a rush to take care of the physical when there is no rush to take care of the mental and emotional?

Journal Prompt #68: Have you ever seen a therapist or counselor? If yes, how has it impacted your life? If not, why not?

Outside of Western medicine, I believe in the power of meditation and working out. I have seen not only the physical but the mental benefits in my body from being active. These are inexpensive and even free ways to help clear your mind and put you in a better mood.

I take daily supplements and also like to take a long bath—and I mean a long hot bath, scorching hot, you can boil a hot potato bath—at least once a week for me to clear my mind. My family knows not to interrupt my bath time.

Maybe you like to take walks alone or read a book or sit in silence. Do your hair or make-up; eat your favorite meal; go out with a friend for coffee, drinks, or dancing; or sit in your car singing 90s R&B songs at the top of your lungs. Also, for me, giving back to those who can never repay me fuels my soul, as well as planning events for my loved ones.

Whatever happiness looks like to you, please find it. When you find it, do that shit. Do that shit as often as possible because you deserve to be happy. You deserve to be healed.

Journal Prompt #69: Do you feel that there is a stigma with seeking professional help for your mental health? How has that impacted the way you see healing?

I learned to put up boundaries. Who has access to my time has changed. Outside of my children, no one gets 24-hour access to me. People who drain my energy, people who are judgemental of me, and people who aren't doing the work for their well-being get their privileges revoked. If I am dealing with my own BS, I do not have the energy to always show up for others 100%, and that is OK. If someone is not OK with me making myself a priority, then access denied. This should go for anyone, including your spouse, your parents, your siblings, and your friends. Know that no one, except for our parents when we are children, owes us anything.

We all know that tomorrow is not promised, but when we take that into account, we realize there is no time to sit around and be angry about things that are beyond our control. Control the controllable. Seeing that has taught me to love a little harder and forgive a little easier.

Journal Prompt #70: What boundaries have you put up in your life, and what boundaries do you still need to establish?

_____

_____

_____

_____

_____

_____

_____

_____

_____

_____

_____

_____

When people show you who they are, believe them and accept them for that.

We only get to make choices for our own lives. We cannot force people into changing, growing, or healing themselves. That is completely on them. We aren't on the same wavelength. We often have to grow apart from those we love the most because sometimes we have to love ourselves more.

Every day get up and remind yourself of who you are. Seriously. Make it a habit.

And at times, you have to learn to be OK with an apology that you'll never receive.

I think that is why I decided not to spend a lot of time talking about the strained relationship I have with my father. Throughout my 30-plus years on earth, he's taken no accountability for not being a father to me and has more often than not shifted the blame to me. At 18, he told me that I was now an adult and needed to get over it. When I was younger, it hurt. Now I realize that he is not self-aware, and gaining such knowledge is something that only he can do for himself.

Ultimately, the people who are supposed to be in your life will be. In relationships, there needs to be reciprocation.

There's work involved in every relationship, whether it is a friendship, a romantic relationship, or your family. There will be work and the people who want to participate. You'll find that you won't have to beg them to. You will not have to plead for them to love you. They just will.

All of us have some type of insecurity. For me, my body image has always sparked huge insecurity. Even though I hate my thick thighs and my big nose, I look at my daughter, whose body shape I can see will be very similar to mine, and I see how insanely beautiful she is. My daughter has the same exact hereditary dark circles I have passed down from my grandmother. I want her to see herself the way I see her, and she cannot if she thinks her mother hates the very body she's inherited. I do not complain about how much I do not like my body in front of her. Instead, I try to praise our body types while also letting her know that having insecurity is 100% normal. It is OK if we do not like something about ourselves. However, it is not my decision, or anyone else's to tell her how she is supposed to feel about her body image.

    Healing is not something that happens automatically or overnight. It is hard work. It takes being honest with yourself, therapy, and confronting your past and present. Healing does not mean you forget. There are some very traumatic things that I am still working through. You may have moments in your life that you are not 100% confident sharing, and that is OK. It is alright to work through things you will not share with everyone, but you do have to do the work to heal yourself. Permit yourself to do the work. Say to yourself, "I get to heal for myself. This is for my benefit."

Journal Prompt #71: Write down your own insecurities. Recognize that it's normal to have insecurities, but you can't allow them to hold you back. What steps can you take to begin healing yours?

Journal Prompt #72: Have you had very traumatic things in your life happen that you are afraid to talk about? Even though it may be hard, what steps can you take to begin healing from them?

_____

_____

_____

_____

_____

_____

_____

_____

_____

_____

_____

_____

_____

AFFIRMATIONS:

- [ ] There is no mountain I cannot climb.
- [ ] I am taking the necessary steps to heal myself.
- [ ] I am strong in my journey.

Set Limits in Your Life

AT THE BLACK GIRLS ROCK AWARDS A FEW YEARS AGO, I was lucky enough to not only sit behind but take a selfie with the one-and-only Angela Bassett. The mother of Trey Styles and Wakanda, Tina Turner, Betty Chavez, Coretta Scott, 9-1-1, the aging queen, and an all-around G.O.A.T, Angela Bassett. As she was receiving the ICON award at the event, she said these words:

> "We all have a purpose. Even if we are still striving to understand what that is…There will be times when you seemingly face insurmountable obstacles, but that is when you dig deep into your soul for the courage and the fortitude to keep going and to never forget that despite life's detours, you are destined for greatness."

I know that some say we shouldn't have to struggle through life to reap a reward, but getting through life without hardships and struggles is just not realistic. It is never going to happen. Your life will never be perfect. We have to learn how to work through things instead of simply trying to get over, by, or past them.

We have to find ways to heal, not just continue to put new bandages on old wounds. We have to heal so that our future trajectory is better than our past.

Another actress who I love is Jenifer Lewis, aka the Mother of Black Hollywood. Such a suitable nickname, as she's played everyone's momma from Tina Turner to *Blackish*. She is a straightforward, tell-it-like-it-is woman. The kind of woman who I deeply admire.

Recently I came across a clip of her saying, "If you sit in shit too long, it stops smelling, so come the fuck outta there."

If I had to sum up this book in one sentence, that would be it. Some of us have become so accustomed to complaining, sulking, to accepting shitty things that they become how we define ourselves and our lives. COME THE FUCK OUTTA THERE! Not one person walking this earth has a perfect life without shit getting in the way. Many have simply learned how to solve the shit and move along.

We have to learn to get out of our own way. Most of us don't want to feel out of control of our lives, so we never leave our comfort zones. We don't want to let others in, so we don't ask for help. Instead, we try to take on everything alone and "solve" all of our own problems unassisted.

This is why we have to heal so that we know when to let others in and so that we don't push away those who have been sent to us as a blessing.

Do things from love. You may not always get it back, but as I always say, your karma is yours, and theirs is theirs.

Speak love and positivity to yourself and over your life. Do it each and every chance you get.

I used to hate looking in the mirror. Now I stop, stare, and say, "Hey you bad bitch, you."

I stopped listening to Drake tell me "no new friends" and made some new ones. I missed my old friends, but I acquired new friends who I have made such deep bonds with over a short amount of time. Ones who support me in my endeavors, who care about what's going on in my life.

I admire friendships that last lifetimes. I have a few, but Stacy from fifth grade is not always supposed to continue with you on your path. There is no room in my life for unsupportive people. What's the use?

One thing that helped me in my healing journey was getting a dog, and you should too! Seriously! Please consider it. Even if you aren't a dog person. I ABSOLUTELY was not. There are even hypoallergenic ones for you all who have allergies. My son had spent 13 years asking for a dog and met with 13 years of "No." Two months after the miscarriage, I gave in, and it has been life-changing. Seriously, Bruno, our 12-pound Cavachon (King Cavalier/Bichon) has been my best medication.

Scientific facts about dogs: They offer unconditional love and support. People with dogs live longer and have lower blood pressure. Dogs alleviate stress. That could be from the multiple daily dog walks, but honestly, I believe it's because the love that dogs give helps our hearts to grow. Maybe just a pet in general, but fish do not give you anything back, and cats can be shady animals. I have had a bunch.

Bruno gives me that same heart-filled love I feel when I think about my grandfather Johnny. It's unconditional love that he does not have to give me, but he does, even when I yell at him for peeing on the floor. He looks up at me with his sad puppy eyes, and it makes my heart melt. When I am sad, it's like he instantly knows and will curl up under me, always making me smile.

Journal Prompt #73: What are some things outside of traditional medicine that aid your healing process? How can you work to incorporate those things even more into your life?

Journal Prompt #74: How do your friends treat you during your hard times? Are there ways they could help you that they haven't? Have you communicated those needs to them?

AFFIRMATIONS:

- [ ] The good energy I put out into the world will come back to me tenfold.
- [ ] I am a good friend.
- [ ] I have everything I need, and that which I don't will come to me.

A Hobby and Self-care

FINDING A HOBBY TO CHANNEL YOUR INNER THOUGHTS into can really help in your healing journey. Art became surprisingly therapeutic for me. I am someone who had a full meltdown in an art class in my 20s because I could not draw.

My niece and daughter love to dance. If my daughter misses a dance rehearsal, she's upset and distraught. It has become not only her passion but her outlet.

Healing and self-care is not a trend, it is not a hashtag, and it is not a pop culture movement. Make it a daily part of your life, like brushing your teeth, walking your dog, or buying yourself a coffee.

Therapy takes time, not a few weeks.

Medication takes time.

Healing takes time.

Heal. Move forward. If the bullshit from the past is still weighing you down, then you aren't healed.

Journal Prompt #75: Write down your hobbies. How can those hobbies become tools on your healing journey?

Journal Prompt #76: How do you practice self-care? If you've fallen behind or don't practice as much, list a few ways you can add self-care to your daily agenda.

AFFIRMATIONS:

- [ ] I am becoming the version of myself I've always wanted to be.
- [ ] I am open to new opportunities.

Fuck That Shit

LETTING GO. SOUNDS A LOT EASIER THAN IT ACTUALLY IS. We are all the villains in someone else's story, and in others, we are the hero. I like to believe them both. Everyone does not get the same version of us. Everyone does not deserve the same version of us. Some people have done us wrong, and we've also hurt others.

Everywhere you go now, you'll hear someone talking about "the vibes." If the vibes are or aren't right, etc. You feel it almost automatically if you aren't "vibing with someone." Trust that shit. I am not into forcing any type of relationship–romantic, friendships, work, platonic, none of it. In the past, I have tried to befriend people who had already had their minds set on not liking me for whatever reason. It was like the ruder they were to me, the more they tried to push me away or the more they shit on me, the harder I tried to show them just how good of a person and friend I was. I wasn't setting boundaries on those who I was allowing into my life.

Changing your mind is not necessarily easy because you cannot control your subconscious. Life happens and pulls us all down at some point. In those moments, allow yourself to feel and move on. Suppressing those feelings is just as harmful as living negatively. Feel them, get through them, and then place them in the box of what was. Practice being intentional about your thoughts, your words, and your actions each and every day.

One day I stopped caring about what others said and thought about me. That shit was making me unhappy. Beyond unhappy, it made me miserable. I was trying so hard to please everyone around me. That is an impossible task for anyone, and if you try, like me you'll get defeated and hate the person who stares back at you in the mirror.

My husband often jokes about me being too real, but it is not that. I just smell BULLSHIT a mile away. Most people aren't ok saying I am fucked up, I am broke, I am broken, I am depressed, I'm overweight, I am a bitch, I am not using my full potential, I need help, I hate my life, I am living a façade, and I am failing, etc. I see it in people. I see them hiding it, and I'm not afraid to say all of the above out loud about myself and if I spot it in others. As you can imagine, being this way hasn't always made me a fan favorite to others, way before reality TV. Most people would rather be fake than be seen for their bullshit. It is the thing about myself that I was constantly trying to hide and change. STOP CALLING PEOPLE OUT ON THEIR BULLSHIT. I couldn't, but once I started to live in my own truth, I lost people and found myself. "If you can't change the people around you, CHANGE THE PEOPLE AROUND YOU."

I have always been afraid of being a failure. Afraid of failing my mom's expectations of me, but more so afraid of failing the little girl I once was who just knew she'd be a success. The girl who knew she would one day take care of her family, support her friends, and make a difference for so many.

At 30-something, I didn't feel like I was her. I was trying incessantly to be her, but it seemed as if no matter how hard I tried, how hard I worked, how good of a mom, wife, and person I was, the universe wasn't reciprocating. I was just that, a failure to myself. I was done. Done trying. I remember praying to God one day in my bedroom like most days, but this day was different. Instead of praying silently in my head, I talked out loud to God. It turned into what seemed like a consistent one-sided conversation, and I was crying while screaming and cursing at God. After what seemed like hours, I looked at myself in the mirror, red-faced, tears streaming, snotty-nosed, and with a pounding headache. I knew at that moment I was defeated. I know I am not perfect, but I support people when they are high and low. I am loyal, I am honest, and I am bitchy, and sarcastic AF. But I do not lie, I do not cheat, and I do not steal–unless it's gloves, alcohol swabs, and cotton balls from the doctor's office. Why wasn't I being rewarded like everyone else seemed to be? There could only be one answer. God either hated me or had forgotten me.

It took me a long time to find myself again and recognize that God (the Universe, Allah, the ancestors, etc.) cannot do all the work. I had to learn to let go and stop begging God to heal me when I wasn't taking all the steps I could to help myself. I needed to learn to start letting go and free myself.

Journal Prompt #77: List events in your life that you need to let go of. Rank them from easiest to hardest, and write down how you can begin to overcome their hold on you.

AFFIRMATIONS:

- [ ] I am letting go of all the things that cannot serve me.
- [ ] I am the hero in the stories of many.

Taking Time Off For Me

YOU WON'T BE POSITIVE ALL THE TIME. IT HAS TO RAIN sometime. And sometimes life will be a fucking monsoon. So when you encounter the "I am always happy and positive" or "Positive vibes only" person, run far, far away from that phony bitch.

If someone I care about has an issue with me or vice versa, I want to talk about it. I like clarity because too often we make up stories and scenarios in our heads that possibly aren't true. I recommend that you do the same. Life is too short to hold long-standing grudges and problems that could be sorted over a coffee or a few lemon-drop martinis.

People too often confuse communication with confrontation. You should always address when you've felt wronged, misunderstood, or disrespected. Learn how to have difficult conversations.

Throughout my life, I have had people who I have loved dearly hurt me, lie to and about me, and more. I have often protected others' reputations by not telling my side of the story. I love the saying "Do not lie about me, and I won't tell the truth about you."

Here is some advice:

Always be an advocate for yourself. Speak up for yourself and set boundaries. This may cause strain or turn uncomfortable in certain relationships. Do it anyway.

Do what the fuck you want to do for and with your life.

Do not fake who you are for anyone.

There will always be someone with something negative to say about your life. Good thing it is your life and not theirs. Fuck those people.

If you always have to be the bigger person, stop hanging with smaller people. We outgrow people.

Tomorrow's not promised. Cuss them out today. (Kidding ...unless you really want to.)

I stopped trying to be a people-pleaser because it wasn't working. It wasn't working for them, and it damn sure wasn't working for me. There are people who I have bent over backward for and they may not have any idea or didn't appreciate it. If you know in your heart you've done the best you can do, and you've been a genuinely good person, then that is all that matters.

People will mistreat you, use you, do you wrong, and judge you. People will talk about you, hate on you, lie about you, make rumors about you, and make you out to be the bad guy.

Everyone is not going to like you, everyone is not going to understand you, and that is OK. You are not here to be everybody's cup of tea. I know I am damn sure not. I don't even really like tea, for real, but I am somebody's shot of vodka.

Stop breaking your own heart by exaggerating your place in other people's lives. There will be people who feel like you are too much, and that is fine. If I am too much for you, you deserve less. It is not selfish to want the same type of love, the same type of support, the same type of whatever that you give to other people returned. Instead of looking for a quantity of people, I wanted quality. Not only those who would support me and vice versa, but those who could teach me, help me, and introduce me to new ways of living, thinking, and seeing life. Find your tribe, find your village, find your circle, and remember that not everyone deserves to sit at your table.

When you aren't invited to the table, do not pull up a chair. Fuck their table. Build your own fucking table.

Journal Prompt #78: Is there someone in your life who you are working to forgive? Why?

AFFIRMATIONS:

☐ My bad days do not define my good days. Just because I have bad days does not mean I am not healing.
☐ I removed bad energy from my life.

Do the Fucking Work

AND ASK FOR HELP.
This was something that I struggled with for so long until ultimately I would become overwhelmed and burned out on my own. I wasn't producing quality work, and my creative juices weren't flowing like they normally would. I was trying to do it all instead of delegating tasks to others. Running a business or even a home takes multiple people with different responsibilities. For me, I am a creative. I have tons of ideas and I'm innovative, but the other side of business was not my strength. Knowing your weaknesses is just as powerful as knowing your strengths. Trying to be the talent, producer, editor, publicist, videographer, photographer, stylist, etc., took away from me producing quality work because I was trying to do every job.

Kevin Hart recently talked about the assumption of ego. Often we do not reach out for help for fear of rejection. We conjure up our own scenarios that others are too busy or that they would never help. You honestly will never know unless you try. The worst that can happen is you get ignored or receive a "No," and then you aren't any worse off than you were. What I have found to be true is that people are more inclined to help you when they see that you are already helping and going above and beyond for your damn self.

You can have a dream, a gift, a passion, and a purpose, BUT if you don't do the work, it's all pointless. You have to DO THE WORK.

In 2020, I made a conscious effort that I had to start doing stuff for myself. I had to stop waiting around for everyone else. Not only that, but I had to learn to do beyond the bare minimum. We often feel like we are doing so much when in reality we aren't. You have to do what not only benefits you but raises you up and holds yourself to a higher standard. You must also recognize the things that are important in your life and make time for them. If it's important to you, then you will find a way. If it is not, then you will find an excuse.

So often nowadays we see everybody posting about their toxic workplace, and so many people want to quit their jobs thinking that self-employment and entrepreneurship are easier. They don't realize that being an entrepreneur is just as demanding, if not more demanding, than a full-time job. When I started my first blog, I probably worked 12 to 16 hours every single day in the beginning. I remember blogging entertainment stories for my first website while I was being induced and in active labor in the hospital with my daughter. Between contractions, I would post on my website, on my social media, and check my email. I did it because I had to, not because I wanted to. I had to work hard for the things I wanted, and that meant there were no days off. There were no sick days. There was no one for me to call when I needed to call out.

I've learned that taking breaks, getting rest, and taking time to reset contributes to my creativity more than I imagined. We live in a world that preaches self-care but also tells us to have no days off. This is why we need a team. This is why we need help. This is why you need to be able to delegate. Stop glamorizing and overworking yourself. Yes, by all means, get that shit done. But also realize that assistance, rest, and resetting are imperative to creativity, productivity, and efficiency.

Issa Rae's character on *Insecure* once said "I just want to fast forward to the part of my life where everything is OK." This is a sentiment that I am sure we all can relate to, but it is not real life. We have to put the work in. It is cliche, but one day you will be so proud of yourself and all the hard work that you put into your success.

Own your shit! Fix your shit!

"If at first you don't succeed, dust yourself off and try again."
— Aaliyah

Journal Prompt #79: Where do you see yourself in five years? In 10 years?

Journal Prompt #80: What steps today will you take to make your dreams a reality?

_____
_____
_____
_____
_____
_____
_____
_____
_____
_____
_____
_____
_____
_____

AFFIRMATION:

☐ Today is a great day to get started.

You Deserve That Shit

I would often feel as though God had forgotten me, or maybe my sole purpose on this earth was to give birth to my two amazing children. Maybe I was only meant to create joy in others' lives by being there for them. I felt this way secretly for many years and then one day, my mindset changed. It was as if God had finally sat me down and said to me, "You are supposed to be happy too. You deserve happiness."

I realized that there were people in my life who I wanted to make proud, my children especially. I wanted them to be just as proud of me as they were of their father. I wanted my husband to be proud of his wife, my mom to be proud of her daughter, and so on. But most importantly. I wanted to make 10-year-old Ashley proud of adult Ashley.

I encourage you to see yourself that way too. Make the people around you proud of you, and make the person who stares at you in the mirror even prouder.

Prioritize whatever you want in your life. The things that fuel your soul, your creativity, and your body are just as important as your education and your job. Doing the shit that makes you happy is valuable. While my youngest niece was entering her senior year of college, she struggled with how to balance work, school, and dance. Someone gave her the advice that dance needed to go on the back burner. My advice to her was absolutely not! We limit ourselves with what we believe about ourselves, so no self-sabotaging.

Do not allow others to strip you of your talents, goals, and the things that truly make you who you are.

No one else gets to tell us what we should prioritize in our lives except for us.

Happiness and success mean something completely different for us all. Too often people correlate the two with money and power, which are made to be our identities. But having money and power isn't the end all be all of happiness, at least not for me. Money is squandered. We see it all the time, those who used to have wealth. And power is often abused. Too often those with power use it to degrade others. Having money and power isn't a negative thing. It's all in how you use them. For me, giving back to the community that I grew up in is a huge dream that I am currently setting in motion. For years I have jokingly told my family and friends that one day I'm going to send them a text saying "Meet me at the airport in an hour. Don't ask questions. Don't bring any bags." A huge part of success and happiness for me is financial freedom so that I can create experiences and memories for those I love.

I often wonder how far ahead I would have been in not just my career but in life if I had not listened to others or if their glass ceilings had not stopped me. I also know it is pointless to sit and cry over should haves, could haves, or would haves. Take that energy and focus on the now and the future. That is what you can take hold of.

Control the controllable.

After having my daughter at 27 years old, I thought to myself. "Damn, I will never have anything else to really celebrate." I had already gotten my first house, I was married, and I had my children. The truth is, we should celebrate more than just the big life events that Hallmark makes cards for. Celebrate the small things. Celebrate fulfilling your dreams and all that you've overcome. Celebrate the person you've become as well as the possibility of a better tomorrow.

Surround yourself with those who you can learn from. Those who push you. Those who give you honest and useful criticism, even when you don't want to receive it. Don't be the oldest, smartest, or most successful in your circle. We are often told that we only live once. I do not find that true. We die once, but every day we are reborn and get a chance to live again. We get a chance to make the lives for ourselves that we want and deserve. Live your dreams, celebrate yourself, control what you can, and let go of what you can't. There is never a better time than now.

Remove the ideal of PERFECTION. No one has it perfect. There is no perfect time or perfect opportunity. It's all in what you do with your time and each opportunity. As cliche as it sounds, what you put in is ultimately what you get out.

I stopped believing that I needed to be the perfect mom, the perfect wife, the perfect whatever. What I needed was to be mentally healthy and happy for myself so that I could love and encourage my kids, husband, and everyone else around me. You must include yourself properly.

I stopped putting a timeline on my success. Just because it took me longer than others doesn't make me a failure. I'm sure you've all seen the meme that says buying a house at 50 is still a success or graduating college at 40 is still a success. It really is. At one point, I decided to put off my career in entertainment because I felt that I was getting too old. I was asked, "Do you want to be 40 with your career or 40 without it." They were right. I want to be 40 with it.

Is there a job that you want but don't think you're qualified for it? Apply anyway.

A guy that you are interested in? Slide in his DM's.

Don't shrink yourself.

Clap for yourself.

See yourself as valuable.

Stand up for yourself.

Never give up.

Stay curious. Stay learning. Stay listening. Never get complacent.

You are more than capable of even your wildest dreams. Change what you believe to be impossible to "it's possible." I encourage you to choose courage over fear every time. I am married to the love of my life, my children are amazing, I am on a successful TV show, and my supporters have grown immensely. I have been given major career opportunities. I've published a damn book! I am currently living inside one of my prayers, and I am sure you are too or one day will be. Take time to show gratitude for these blessings. Reward and applaud yourself for all achievements, no matter how minor they may seem to you.

I am thankful to myself that I never decided to have a Plan B or a backup plan, as many told me that I should have. My life is exactly where it should be when it should be.

Tell yourself:

I am very intentional about my mental health. "No" and "OK" are full sentences.

I am very intentional about my self-awareness. I know exactly who I am.

I am very intentional about my happiness.

Be proud of who you are instead of ashamed of who you aren't. While writing this journal, there were times I felt apprehensive about sharing certain details of my life. What would my mom say? How would my husband feel? What will my kids think of me, not to mention the readers and critics!?!? LAWD! The court of public opinion is tough. It can beat you down and judge you tremendously for sharing your truth. But what I know is that all of us fall short at times. All of us have something in our lives that is less than stellar, all of us have a story, and those are the things that make us who we are. Beyond that, I know that God knows exactly who I am. I can't hide from Him. And I know myself. I know who I am wholeheartedly, the good, the bad, and the in-between. I'm not out here pretending to be someone I am not. This is the life that I have led. And I am proud of the road I am currently traveling in my exploration of life.

I now acknowledge the GREEN flags in my life. There is so much greatness happening around me, for me, and within me. Earlier I stated that we are all currently living inside of one of our blessings and that we should be grateful for these blessings. To really realize these blessings, invite your past to the party in your present. Ten-year-old me knew that one day this life I am currently living would be here. She's proud. Twenty-something me, the one who had extensive doubt about if my dreams of happiness and success would ever come to fruition, is so elated that she has finally come out of that deep dark hole.

Allow yourself to be happy, to love, to be loved, and to experience all the joy that you feel. When you are feeling that happiness, joy, and success, yell it out so that everyone can hear it. Don't hold your joy in. You came a long way to get to it. Praise yourself and watch just how much more greatness starts to flow your way.

The secret that we all are so desperately searching for isn't a secret at all. The answer is that you cannot just be willing, able, and motivated. You have to be disciplined beyond belief. There are ultimately only two options in life: Do that shit or don't. You have to do that shit on the days that you are tired, on the days that you are sad, on the days that you are grieving, on the days that you are lonely, on the days that you are broke, and every day in between. You have to get the fuck up and do it!

As my husband likes to proudly say, "HARD WORK, DEDICATION, AND CONSISTENCY."

What's meant for you will happen. It is time for you to take control of your life.

My mom was right all those years ago. I was living in a fantasy land, and I still am. It is called Ashleyland, the happiest place on earth, and I love it here.

This is not the end…it's just the beginning!

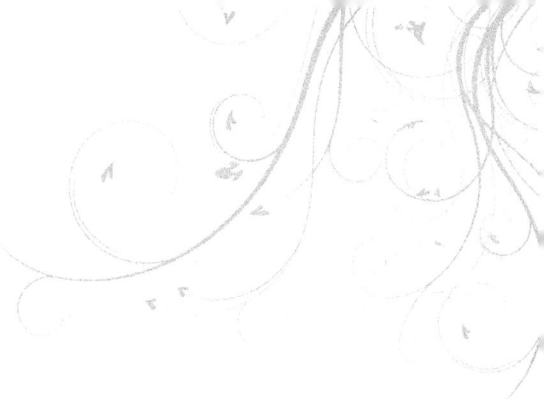

Epilogue

JOURNEYS ARE HARD, BUT THE MOST DIFFICULT PART IS THE beginning. As I began my own journey, I had to learn the hard way that the only way out is through. That reality came crashing down on me in waves of depression and early life crisis. I wasn't who I wanted to be and I was nowhere near happy. Once I realized that I needed to change, I began my journey.

It has been tough, the roads are sometimes ragged and rough. There are many days where I feel like giving up. Where I stop and feel as if the ground is falling out from under me. I am here to say that no matter how dark your world is, no matter how scary the start of the journey is, there is always light at the end of the tunnel.

Do that shit and do it for *you*. Allow yourself to be the center of your own world, even if only for a day.

Work on yourself and don't half ass it. Manifest your dreams into reality. Work hard so that one day you can look back at the journey you took and be proud of the person you have become.

Your story is going to be a good one.

I want to share some quotes, mantras, movie lines, and songs that I live by. They are below.

DO THAT SH!T

"There are people who have money and people who are rich."
— Coco Chanel

"Remind yourself. Nobody's built like you, You design yourself."
— Jay Z

"When I let go of what I am, I become what I might be." – Lao Tzu

"A grateful heart is a magnet for blessings"
— Shakira Maria

"We cannot become what we want to be by remaining what we are."
— Max Depree

"Take the craziest dream you ever had and go after it. Make it a reality. I don't want you to dream, I want you to do."
— Puff Daddy

"You should aspire to have the richest life you can get in terms of fulfillment, happiness, and peace."
— Kimora Lee Simmons

"Let's not be mediocre in our greatness"
— Lauryn Hill

"You can't just sit there and wait for people to give you that golden dream. You've got to get out there and make it happen for yourself."
— Diana Ross

"Be nice to yourself… It's hard to be happy when someone is mean to you all the time."

— Christine Arylo

"I believe that if you'll just stand up and go, life will open up for you."

— Tina Turner

"Happiness is not something that just comes to you. It's an active process."

— Kate Hudson

"If everything was perfect, you would never learn and you would never grow."

— Beyoncé

"Do what you were born to do. You have to trust yourself."

— Beyoncé

"I will not let anyone walk through my mind with dirty feet."

— Gandhi

"If I give them the power to feed me, I also give them the power to starve me."

— Steve Maraboli

"Don't try to lessen yourself for the world; Let the world catch up to you."

— Beyoncé

"I ain't scare of s***. I will always speak on how I feel I'll be damn if fame and other people have me being a slave of my own thoughts."
— Cardi B

"Your power is in your individuality, in being exactly who you are."
— Jennifer Lopez

"Ignore the glass ceiling and do your work. If you're focusing on the glass ceiling, focusing on what you don't have, focusing on the limitations, then you will be limited."
— Ava Duvernay

"If somebody says no, you're asking the wrong person."- Kris Jenner
"You have to believe in yourself when no one else does."
— Serena Williams

"Take a chance and never look back. Never have regrets, just lessons learned."
— Kim Kardashian

"We don't back off obstacles and tough situations, we use them to make us stronger."
— Jada Pinkett Smith

"If you can do what you do best and be happy, you are further along in life than most people."
— Leonardo DiCaprio

"Success is only meaningful and enjoyable if it feels like your own."
— Michele Obama

"I refuse to accept other people's ideas of happiness for me. As if there's a one size fits all standard for happiness."

— Kanye West

"If you do what you've always done, you'll get what you've always gotten."

— Tony Robbins

"There is only one way to avoid criticism: Do nothing, say nothing, and be nothing."

— Aristotle

"You get what you settle for."

— Thelma and Louise

"No one is immune to the trials and tribulations of life."

— Martin Lawrence

"Doing the best at this moment puts you in the best place for the next moment."

— Oprah Winfrey

"Be thankful for what you have; you'll end up having more. If you concentrate on what you don't have, you will never, ever have enough."

— Oprah Winfrey

"Turn your wounds into wisdom."

— Oprah Winfrey

"It's nice to look back on your life and see things as lessons, and not regrets."

— Rihanna

"Forever, I'm that girl."

— Beyoncé

"Do what you gotta do so you can do what you wanna do."

— Denzel Washington

"You can't make decisions based on fear and the possibility of what might happen."

— Michelle Obama

"Cause everybody dies but not everybody lives."

— Drake

www.ingramcontent.com/pod-product-compliance
Lightning Source LLC
Chambersburg PA
CBHW050246010526
44107CB00003B/203